SACRED
SEXUAL UNION

•

"In her book *Sacred Sexual Union,* Anaiya Sophia asks a question of timeless importance: 'Is sacred union real?' It's clear she has also lived the question, in both ordinary and extraordinary ways, making this more than an ordinary book, but a pure expression of the search for the Beloved. You'll find yourself on every page, since, after all, the Beloved is within you."

JAMES F. TWYMAN, PEACE TROUBADOUR
AND AUTHOR OF THE BESTSELLING *THE MOSES CODE*

"*Sacred Sexual Union* is the most comprehensive, insightful, and inspiring work by Anaiya Sophia thus far! From the wounds of love to womb healing and *hieros gamos,* Anaiya takes readers on a healing journey deep within to answer questions about the true nature of love and what life within sacred union looks like. Pulling from great ancient records, this mystical journey connects us to the true depth of ourselves, our twin soul, and the all-encompassing love from the divine. This is a must-read for any and all on the true love, sacred union path."

HEATHER STRANG, AUTHOR OF
THE QUEST: A TALE OF DESIRE & MAGIC

"*Sacred Sexual Union* is a beautiful recognition and celebration of sacred union as the path to God, herself. We have been looking for God alone in meditation forever. She is not there. She is on the bridge between two hearts, awakened and illuminated by their shared breath, conscious intentionality, and authentic self-revealing. Through the merging of two willing souls, the gateway opens to the everything. There is such magic in these pages."

JEFF BROWN, AUTHOR OF *SOULSHAPING*

"Regardless of your path, *Sacred Sexual Union* will help you discover fascinating ways to delve deeply into the mysterious crucible of love. Anaiya's passionate guide takes you through and beyond the surface of physical love, where you can explore the magical realms of sexual union."

AMARA CHARLES, AUTHOR OF
THE SEXUAL PRACTICES OF QUODOUSHKA

SACRED SEXUAL UNION

The Alchemy of Love, Power, and Wisdom

ANAIYA SOPHIA

Destiny Books

Rochester, Vermont • Toronto, Canada

Destiny Books
One Park Street
Rochester, Vermont 05767
www.DestinyBooks.com

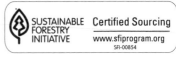

Text stock is SFI certified

Destiny Books is a division of Inner Traditions International

Library of Congress Cataloging-in-Publication Data
Sophia, Anaiya, 1969–
  Sacred sexual union : the alchemy of love, power, and wisdom / Anaiya Sophia.
    p. cm.
  Includes index.
  ISBN 978-1-62055-007-6 (pbk.) — ISBN 978-1-62055-149-3 (e-book)
  Summary: "Experience the orgasmic rapture of Sacred Union with your Twin
Soul and the Divine"—Provided by publisher.
  1. Sex—Religious aspects. 2. Love—Religious aspects. I. Title.
  BL65.S4S67 2013
  204'.46—dc23

                                               2012035076

Printed and bound in the United States by Lake Book Manufacturing, Inc.
The text stock is SFI certified. The Sustainable Forestry Initiative® program
promotes sustainable forest management.

10 9 8 7 6 5 4 3 2 1

Text design and layout by Virginia Scott Bowman
This book was typeset in Garamond Premier Pro and Gill Sans with Cochin and
Trajan Pro used as display typefaces
Illustrated by Cathy Hilton, www.cathyhiltonartisan.co.uk

Poems on pages 1, 41, 113, and 128 from "Ritual of the Bridal Chamber," by
Bishop Rosamonde Miller, reprinted by permission of the author.

To send correspondence to the author of this book, mail a first-class letter to the
author c/o Inner Traditions • Bear & Company, One Park Street, Rochester, VT
05767, and we will forward the communication, or contact the author directly at
www.anaiyasophia.com or **www.pilgrimageoflove.com**.

אֲנִי לְדוֹדִי וְדוֹדִי לִי

I am my beloved's, and my beloved is mine.

SONG OF SOLOMON 6:3

This book is dedicated to those who have the eyes to see and the ears to hear.

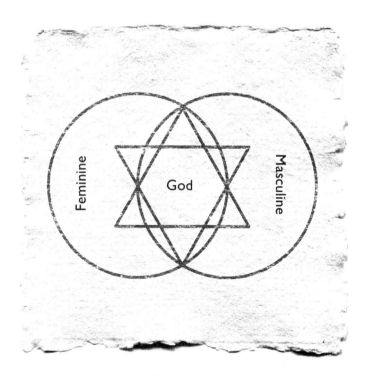

Vesica Piscis

CONTENTS

PART ONE
Sacred Sexuality
The First Trimester

PART TWO

Emotional Intimacy

The Second Trimester

PART THREE

Soul Consciousness

The Third Trimester

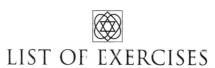

LIST OF EXERCISES

I Am the Black Thunder

I am the black mountain, and the sound of my thunder
   welcomes You
I am the seer of this world, all that is seen and unseen is
   witnessed by Me
I am that joy that swells in your heart at the close encounter
   of my countenance
I am the reaching, the longing, and the final embrace

You belong to Me, and I belong to You
Bathe in my waters, and surrender to my tranquil waves
I am calling You throughout time and space
Rip through the veils of this world and glimpse my face
Gather your Soul and surge onward to our Destiny
An unknowable knowingness is breathing endlessly

Words drop to their knees in exasperation
Offerings crumble and whither
Prayers wash through the ocean and dissolve
Only the Soul full fire reaches my shores

Crash your ego upon the alter of Love
Only those as gentle as the dove, shall rest within Me
I will plunge into your truth and pull out the worms
Until You and I are One
I am the Thunder of the Black Mountain

ANAIYA SOPHIA

PREFACE

It all began on the steps of the Basilica of the Sacred Heart in Paris, also known as the Sacré-Coeur, when at the tender age of seven I miraculously laid eyes on the beloved masquerading as a beggar. In that timeless moment that continues to live on with my every breath, I saw the original creation and our fall from the metaphorical Garden of Eden. I saw the timeline and process of our separation from God. As I continued to look into his eyes, I sensed the overwhelming love of God pouring out of this man toward me. Within his glance I was able to connect with the other half of my soul. Words could never truly reveal the enormity of that moment, except to say that it ignited a longing and a desire to find him on Earth again. That meeting birthed an undeniable force within me that searched for those eyes everywhere. This event marked the beginning of my pilgrimage of love. I read countless books and sat at the feet of many a spiritual teacher. I simply had to know the way of being able to reunite with my soul half here on Earth and what that would look like.

This burning desire consumed me, and I found no joy outside its flames.

Days turned into months; as months became years an inexhaustible desire to know and to experience the fullness of love grew in me. It was tangibly felt in the parchments of Rumi's poetry and the intoxicating letters from

Saint Clair of Assisi, describing her untamable love of God. What was this longing that I so desperately recognized and hungered to follow?

I ached to become love and live a life that was sincere, pure, and true. Above and beyond that desire was my steadfast intention to meet my soul half and to begin our soul reunification process together. I discovered processes and sex magic rituals based on ancient practices from Egypt and Sumeria that spoke of soul union. This was close, but was not it. I briefly explored Tantra and its various forms of sacred sexuality—this absolutely was not it. I knew there was more, and that something contained a depth of consistent being that inspired me.

I had now reached a point in my life where all seeking had to cease, and instead I had to begin to live what was already known within me. I had to discover and live my longing to its fullness, to tirelessly forge my own self in the fires of creation and bring forth my soul half with the intention to carve open the soul reunification process for ourselves and others. Knowing with unwavering certainty that this work would become my soul contribution in this lifetime, I was willing to bleed, sweat, cry, and claw my way toward the authentic answer. Was there an alchemical process that soul halves had to experience in order to reunify, or was this just a fantastical story?

I had to know—was sacred union real?

Is there a path that leads to our true inheritance, where a man and a woman can walk together, hand in hand, toward God as a means of attaining soul reunion? Was there a path where mortals in the past have tasted the euphoria of uniting with the Divine through relationship with their beloved? Could there be a process that surpasses the teacher-student dynamic of a more traditional spiritual path, a gateway of evolution that is available for all despite worldly limitations? Could there be a process in which the only currency that is required is the true and relentless desire to know God by loving ever deeper?

This was and is my only contemplation.

☩

Over the past twenty years I have passionately pieced together the conscious elements of sacred union, also known as *hieros gamos,* or the sacrament of the bridal chamber. These terms refer to the sacred marriage between two divinities, a human being and God, or two human beings; it is the ultimate alchemy of forces that harmonize polar opposites, dissolving all duality.

Is it possible that sacred sexual union, based upon the conscious application of love, power, and wisdom, could be the path to attain Christhood? Can hormonally driven sex be preventing men and women from rediscovering their innate nondual perception?

Perhaps the only way to discover the truth is to attempt to re-create the experience of the sacrament of the bridal chamber for ourselves. Within this book you will discover not only the entrance to such a process but also a guiding light that can only come from integrated direct experience. My studies have included kundalini yoga, universal Kabbalah, the Egyptian Mystery traditions, sexual shamanism, gnostic mysticism, and Christianity. My initiations included healing myself from cervical cancer using the ancient methods of the Holy Order of Mary Magdalene and reclaiming my own power and voice in the world after hitting rock bottom on every level imaginable.

Today I tell a different story. Today I am filled with an insatiable spiritual fire urging me to discover and awaken those who hear the call and feel the same longing to return once again, to be consciously chosen and entered into in the process of sacred union.

To all of you who thirst for the truth, know that the preparatory stages of sacred union are intended to be one of the most profoundly transformative periods of your lifetime. This path is for the courageous of heart and requires a full commitment to show up and give 100 percent to its process. This is not for those of you who may be seeking better sex or a more fulfilling relationship. This is not a practice or a ıal; it is a deep and consuming way of life. It requires everything, all that you are and all that you shall become.

With this work we can sometimes make the mistake of imagining that we are preparing for our twin soul (soul half), that we are clearing the path for him or her to enter. We are not clearing a path but rather allowing the magnetic pull of our soul to draw our being back together. Our twins and ourselves are not separate. They are our other half. What we do to engage ourselves affects them. The more we live our true desires and passions, the closer they shall come to us. The more we become the wholeness of ourselves, the more undeniable the pull toward us becomes.

This work transforms the entirety of our being on Earth (both halves) to reflect the true and lasting beauty of our soul. Every meticulous inner movement of discomfort in its varying forms is used as an ally to highlight areas where a state of separation still exists. When two people commit to this process, they will experience a crucible of alchemical friction that creates the vibrational frequency required to responsibly embody the luminescence of true Christ consciousness.

This book is dedicated to the scorching longing you feel within you to open to this sacred mystery and embody its rapturous juice with your everyday life. My desire has always been to experience what the Persian poet Rumi and his spiritual instructor Shams lived, and to then share and support those of you who hunger to do the same. I know that this love is not the privilege of the saints, sufis, or other mystical beloveds bound by text and legend. This divine love of God is waiting for us all to say yes and to joyfully embrace it with our every breath as we surrender our lives at God's feet.

This book is centered on the threefold flame of power (sacred sexuality), love (emotional intimacy), and wisdom (soul consciousness). The threefold flame is at the sacred heart of Christ consciousness and is the central pillar of all alchemy.

Sacred union is an experiential journey and process. For a complete understanding and more information about this unfolding journey, please visit my websites:

www.anaiyasophia.com

Here you will find my books, worldwide gatherings, online courses, transformational processes, and downloadable albums, articles, and meditations. You can also watch my YouTube videos on the Anaiya Sophia Channel. You are welcome to visit my home and temple, the New Renaissance, in Chalabre, France—a creative and mystical arts space dedicated to the Christ lineage mysteries and situated between Montségur and Rennes-le-Château.

I move forward with trust and consciousness.

This Dance

We have come to be danced
Not the "I am pretty, pick me, pick me!" dance
But the claw our way back into the belly
Of the sacred, sensual animal dance
The unhinged, unplugged, cat is out of its bag dance
The holding of the precious moment in the palms
Of our hands and feet dance.

We have come to be danced
Not the nice, invisible, self-conscious little shuffle
But the matted hair flying, voodoo mama
Shaman shaking, ancient bones dance
The strip us from our prison, returning our wings
Sharpening our claws and tongues dance
That shed dead cells as we slip into
The luminous skin of love dance.

We have come to be danced
Where the kingdoms collide
In the cathedral of flesh
To burn back into the light
To unravel, to play, to fly, to pray
To root in skin sanctuary
We have come to be danced!
We have come . . .

JEWEL MATHIESON
(WWW.JEWELM.NET)

ACKNOWLEDGMENTS

To my parents, Dinah and Patrick Cuddihy, for taking me to Sacré-Coeur in Paris when I was seven years old—upon those steps I saw the face of love, and not for one moment did I ever stop looking for the source of that unspeakable glance—thank you both so deeply for seeding within me this inextinguishable fire of love and for bringing me into this world in the first place.

To my passionate and magical midwives and editors, Jenna Paulden and Heather Strang, who have always stood beside me on this quest and whose support I shall remember until the end of time.

To my dear friend and fellow pilgrim Cathy Hilton, who almost overnight miraculously produced all the illustrations for this book.

To my beloved friends Carolyn Billingham, Oshun Du Bellay, and Nicolya Christi, who have my back in every dimension as much as I have theirs. Throughout all time and space, I shall love you.

To the men and women who walk this path beside me, offering crystal-clear reflections, sincere friendship, and devotion to the ever deepening—there are way too many to mention, but you know who you are.

To Rumi and Shams, who always ignited my faith on days when I had given up.

To all my teachers on the path of love, I send you unspeakable gratitude.

Every word that has been written and all the spaces in between are dedicated to my beloved, Luc Tibor, who walks beside me on this journey—the one who inspires me to live and breathe the love, truth, and humility of our soul.

To Jon Graham, Meghan MacLean, and the team at Inner Traditions, who supported and manifested this book into the world. Thank you for making the process so graceful and easy, it is a delight to work and share with you all.

May you all know how deeply you have touched me and that this touch reverberates throughout the entire cosmos.

INTRODUCTION

I am holding you and not letting you go.
Hear me you who call.
Hear me, and do not turn your face from me at any place
  or at any time.
I am she who gives her life to the depth of matter.
I prepare the Bread and Wine in you that you may
  remember the Spark of Life.

HOLY SOPHIA'S WORDS,
FROM "RITUAL OF THE BRIDAL CHAMBER,"
BY BISHOP ROSAMONDE MILLER

We are entering a new renaissance. A time where (mostly) women and a growing number of courageous men are carrying the mantel of the Divine Feminine in a powerful and creative way. You shall know these ones by the wisdom streaming through their eyes, the power pulsing from their wombs and *haras,* and the love pouring through their hearts and souls. They have been shaped and carved by life, by living fully, dying consciously, and loving tremendously. They restore their honorable power by retrieving their own fragmented parts. They blaze with the love of the Divine. Like comets, they sweep into your life, reminding you of what it means to be truly *alive,* to be aflame with the bridal chamber, where matter and spirit become one. They house the greatest secrets of all time in their touch, their words, their glance, and their eternal presence.

Through the mists of our time, true kings and queens are being born. And in their wake—a legacy of elegance, sovereignty, and almighty compassion.

There has always been a hidden pathway and secret ritual that brings forth the reunion of soul halves (twin souls). This profoundly rich work once belonged to the legacy and legends of the Grail lineage, also known as the Rose Line. The priestesses of this lineage knew how this infinite mystery was lying dormant inside each and every one of us and that it was their divine purpose to awaken the spark of life from its slumber. They knew about the seed within us that contains the living memory of a mysterious doorway that leads two souls into their original state of creation, where they were as one before their separation.

Not only is it a doorway that lovers ecstatically merge in to, it is also a dimensional space where a glimpse of reunified soul can be tangibly felt. In some of the more ancient gnostic scriptures we are told that God has also become separated into two parts, one masculine and one feminine. We are told that the sacred union process in which a man and a woman merge into one is additionally a way for God the Father to reunite with God the Mother. As the story continues, we are told that when God the Father experiences the fullness of his reunion with the Mother, there is an almighty blessing bestowed upon the two human beings in rapturous union. This explosion of orgasmic light from their Creator brings forth the fullness of their soul union potential. As with all gnostic texts, nothing means anything *unless* it is directly experienced.

To enter through this doorway we have to become lovers with a capital L. Lovers of life, beauty, music, art, the mystery, and, above all, Love. We have to engage with ourselves fully, as we earnestly follow our true passions and desires. In order to attract our soul half, we have to awaken, live, and thrive off our own essence. We have to love our lives so deeply that the magnetic energies of the soul start to draw its twin into its physical proximity.

Throughout the ages, sacred union has been associated with many other names, such as hieros gamos (holy marriage) in Christianity, yab-yum in Tibetan Buddhism, sacred marriage in the Kabbalah, and, in some ways, Tantra in Hinduism. But none of these fully encompass what I am referring to. I am speaking of an authentic and pure way of living that supports the soul reunification process between soul halves. This is not a singular form of sacred sexuality, meditation, prayer, or intimacy. It is all of those consistently combined as a way to progress in love toward God.

As we look back in history, we catch glimpses of this sacred union rapture and no doubt experience a quiet despair as we face the emptiness within our own lives today. Where is this passion of which the drunken love poet Rumi speaks? How did King Solomon become filled with the spirit of eternal wisdom after spending one lunar cycle with the Queen of Sheba? What is this story of God the feminine (Sophia), who forsook her divinity to save her children on Earth, and the fiery longing of God the Logos to find and reunite with her? How come the ancients knew of this story and covered all their temple walls with images to symbolize the reunion of the masculine and feminine? If we are made in God's image, then it stands to reason that God is both male and female. Two aspects in one entity. In my conclusion we, God's creation, must also be the same.

Sacred union is the alchemical process that reveals this truth: that in our original creation there were two aspects in the one soul and for some mysterious reason we separated and became two individual halves. It is by the consistent living of sacred union that twin souls can and shall coalesce with the humble reliance on God to help them overcome every and all obstacles.

The Egyptian and gnostic scriptures as well as the delectable Sufi poetry allow us to experience God in a fresh, new way. And the more we read, the more we understand that *their* God was very different from the one that is etched into the fabric of our psyches. Their God is full of longing, yearning, and rapture to dance and play with its human creation. It longs and aches for us as much as we long and ache for it. Their God is sensual, rich, and touchable; their God is both feminine and masculine; and even wilder still, their God comes alive inside them, making its presence known in an undeniable way. Then it became clear. Sacred union can only be experienced if one carries within love, surrender, and openness to the fullness of life in all its expressions. It is this love that is the energy, fuel, and movement that catalyzes the energies that will explode our sense of consciousness from the confines of being human to that of being ecstatically and intimately in love with our Creator and our creation.

When you love with all of your existence, there is no fear, no limits, and no such thing as boundaries. When you crack open the shell of being human, there is a wealth of energy that can be both unshackled and harnessed for something far greater than merely existing. For maybe the first time—like virgins—we touch and taste the original desire our Creator has carried in its heart; its longing for our true purpose.

Take just a moment, if you will, to contemplate this notion of a masculine God longing, aching, and yearning to reunite with his feminine essence inside our heart, body, and soul. We will be going into much more detail with this prime gnostic teaching throughout the pages of this book. So it's essential for you to begin to sit with this now and start to feel these energies of longing, gratitude, and rapture within you.

The ways and means of not only practically unifying with your twin soul but also the fullness of God shall become known to you through this book. It has been my ardent and often harrowing journey to find out how the soul reunification happens and what the obstacles are along the way. Within this journey we shall continue to discover countless forms of higher states of union—the higher we go, the subtler the experience. Once you surrender to the inherent pull of the soul to come together, then you realize that you have just tapped in to the greatest forces ever known. Like giant cosmic magnets, their power lies within their destiny to reunite in sacred union. It has been my personal journey to find the way to piece the puzzle back together, and even I do not have the end result. All I have is how and why. You have to take this further—as I sense in the innermost aspect of my being that each and every one of us has the opportunity to go far beyond what I have experienced and written about.

I knew that sacred union was not a mystical meditation or yogic state. My soul endlessly reminded me of how this experience happens *inside* the body and becomes part of the fabric of one's day-to-day life. Somehow we have to awaken these energies inside our body, as everything exists within us. Only through this awakening process will we recognize and remember our twin soul, the one with whom it is our destiny to reunite.

I was being led to create a picture, a map, and a process.

* First, you prepare: sacred work
* Second, you meet: the glance (*nazar*)
* Third, you initiate: the kiss (*nashakh*)

Following the principles of the threefold flame (power, love, and wisdom—the pillar stone of all alchemy), I knew that the foundation stones of sacred union would involve the uniting and merging of sexuality, the heart, and consciousness. I also knew that this foundational process requires a nine-month preparatory process based on the three trimesters of a human pregnancy: three months spent working with sacred sexuality, three months spent working on emotional intimacy, and another three months spent predominantly on soul consciousness.

Toward the very end of this book I share with you the tenth month, the final piece of the puzzle. Like the tenth sphere in the Tree of Life, herein lies the mystery. This final process is an alchemical gateway where this book gets discarded and the fullness of love takes over. This tenth insight is not something that you learn but rather something you live. It must be restated here that this ritualistic process weaves together the very fabric of one's being, hence it can only ever be done with your twin soul (more about that in the next chapter). However, embarking upon this journey will powerfully reveal who is and who is not your soul half. The clearer you become, the more you will know the truth of your twin soul. This is not a process to achieve great sex, have a romantic love affair, or gain cosmic powers. This is a fundamental upheaval of your entirety that forever alters your existence. No stone is left unturned as you seek for every strand of fear and distrust that attempts to sabotage the process.

In the New Age spiritual market we read about the twin flames, their ecstatic coming together, and how their great love births the new era of humanity. The problem with the New Age philosophy is its empty promises and sweet-as-honey perspective. Where we are going is real and deep and requires us to roll up our egoic sleeves as we get down and dirty. This is not a part-time or weekend fancy; this hunger for our soul half and its reunification consumes our lives and then begs for more.

I am often asked, "But how do we know if we have met our twin soul?" This truly is the million-dollar question. Luckily, scattered throughout the stories of sacred union, we occasionally find pieces of treasure that attempt to answer some of our very natural human questions. These are the nuggets for which I have spent my life searching. There is a part in the *Pistis Sophia* where we learn that Sophia (feminine aspect of God) has lost her sight since falling to Earth and that she cannot see the Logos (masculine aspect of God) standing before her. The only way that she knows it's him is by her ability to *feel*. This is a very important clue. You shall know your twin soul by the way he or she makes you feel. There will be a timeless quality of deep trust, brother/sister love, passion, longing, gratitude, and unspeakable happiness. When you feel the qualities of "father, brother, son, and husband" in the masculine and "mother, sister, daughter, and wife" in the feminine—pay attention!

The beloved (the living prayer within your soul—both halves) is an inexhaustible force of love that is absolutely destined to reunite in exquisite totality. It will not and cannot falter as it ravishes the very idea of entering into the fabric of your life. Death does not stop this process. The moment you dedicate your life in devotion to know this love, it comes. The very mystery of whispering this yes to sacred union sets the wheels in motion for the beloved to appear and dance with you.

To open the doorway of the beloved and into the fathomless dimensions of love and unspeakable communion with our Creator takes a sincere and pure prayer. This is the initiation of our birthright that will allow us to step in to the fullness of our authentic glory. And this initiation is to be found within these pages.

ANCIENT AND MODERN EXAMPLES

Throughout ancient texts and poetry and many modern-day films there are two patterns that stand out so clearly above all the rest. First is how the twinned lovers become, almost overnight, great kings and queens, rulers of abundant and prosperous civilizations, and/or creators of some wondrous breakthrough in our human history.

Second, it is the women who are the ones who lead and initiate the sacred union process (the magical ingredient) that saves the day. It seems to me that this message of the feminine leading the way is yet another reflection of the Divine Feminine resurgence that we are seeing everywhere these days. It is true to say that the house of relationship sits within the realm of the feminine principle (in both men and women) and that this process begins, is guided by, and comes to fruition through the feminine essence.

Let us now look at some of the historical examples of human beings who have entered into mystical union to see whether we can spot any further patterns and clues about sacred union.

King Solomon and the Queen of Sheba

The best-known historical example of such a sacred marriage is between King Solomon and the Queen of Sheba. The Queen of Sheba traveled from her homeland to meet Solomon to perform the hieros gamos with him, otherwise known as being together in the bridal chamber. She had heard of King Solomon and was moved by the very mention of his name. Upon seeing one another they both knew that they were twin souls.

The Queen of Sheba could never marry Solomon as they were rulers of different lands, and in those days you married within your own kingdom. She was, however, a high priestess and knew the rites and rituals of hieros gamos. She was able to spend one lunar cycle with Solomon before having to return to her homeland. Once the queen left, King Solomon *then* became a legendary king renowned for his wisdom. As a result of sacred union King Solomon was initiated into the next quantum level of his destiny. Basking in the glory of their union, King Solomon wrote his most famous poem the "Song of Songs," dedicated to the Queen of Sheba. This poem is one of hundreds of attempts to capture the essence of his eternal love for his soul half and sister bride.

Isis and Osiris

In *The Passion of Isis and Osiris,* a book written by Jean Houston an internationally renowned philosopher, psychologist, and explorer of world myth, we get to read how Isis and Osiris sought reunion within each one of us. In ancient Egypt the marriage between Isis and Osiris was considered the sacred union of heaven and Earth, of yin and yang, of the feminine and the masculine principles.

In the story of Isis and Osiris we learn that it was Isis who was able to put Osiris back together again after he had been torn into pieces and scattered by his evil brother, Set. When at last all the parts had been assembled, Isis made Osiris into the first Egyptian mummy. She then used her powerful magic to breathe new life into Osiris, and in doing so she was able to conceive the child Horus. In time Osiris became the king of the Land of the Dead, while Horus fought against his uncle Set, won back his father's throne, and became the living king of Egypt. During the time of Isis and Osiris, the fall of Egypt occurred.

El and Asherah

In the ancient Hebrew Bible we learn of El and Asherah, our heavenly Father and Mother (God in its masculine and feminine principles). It was the desire of El and Asherah to experience their great and holy love in a more expressive physical form and to share that blessing with all the children they would create. For the very first time we hear how the divine ritual of sacred union was created. Like Sophia and the Logos, El and Asherah longed for all their creations to carry their inexhaustible love within them for this was their light and their power. They desired for the whole of creation to be alive and vibrating with their longing to merge. Therefore they created an alchemical ritualistic process wherein the essence of El and Asherah entered into the man and woman who not only granted full permission but also wholeheartedly sought that essence.

Sophia and the Logos

In *Pistis Sophia,* a gnostic text, we discover a similar story, that of Sophia and the Logos, the masculine and feminine aspects of God that long to discover one another and merge again here on Earth. In this book we learn that Sophia relinquished her divinity to attend to the pain and suffering of all her children on Earth.

What happened and was not planned for was the fall. Sophia became trapped on Earth because of the enormity of density that had built up, and suddenly she lost her way back home. God the Father did not know where Sophia had gone and over time fell into a painful depression. In the end he decided to create the Logos, the light of God's love, and sent him forth to seek out Sophia. In this study we come to understand that Sophia and the Logos have been seeking one another since the beginning of time, and until each and every one of us falls into ecstatic union with God, they will not stop being magnetized toward one another.

Jesus Christ and Mary Magdalene

The most recent historical couple to enter into sacred union is Jesus Christ and Mary Magdalene. In the hidden gospels of Mary Magdalene, Philip, and Thomas, we discover passages that clearly state that Jesus and Mary were married, and on their wedding day they entered into hieros gamos, or the bridal chamber.

It was because of their mystical union that Jesus Christ was able to live through the Crucifixion. We also see that Mary did not leave the side of Jesus throughout the whole of the Good Friday ordeal and that she was present for every twist and turn that unfolded. Like Isis, she administered the death rites and prepared his body for the resurrection. Throughout the pages of the Gospel of Philip we learn that it was Mary Magdalene who received the majority of Christ's apparitions and mystical teachings once he was resurrected. It's interesting to note that toward the end of Jesus's ministry "he appointed seventy-two disciples, and sent them out, two by two to go and spread the good news" (Luke 10).

Nowhere in the Bible does it say that these disciples were pairs of men. Could it be that these disciples were in fact beloved twin soul couples and the way was in fact an initiatory pathway based on love, power, and wisdom—the very same path that is touched on here?

And so we see a pattern forming: the emergence of a lineage of sister priestesses, the true meaning of resurrection, everlasting life, and a love that is truly eternal and continuous. Osiris, El, King Solomon, the Logos, and Jesus Christ all became architects of our known universe. Their queens knew how to perform the hieros gamos and the alchemical ways to harness the powers to perform the rites of resurrection. In addition there was almost always a great fall of a corrupt civilization along with huge geographical changes across the planet that took place once these twin souls merged in sacred union.

Modern Examples

When we look at our culture's modern-day examples of beloveds in sacred union, we see similar patterns playing out, with exactly the same outcome.

Neo and Trinity from *The Matrix* witness the fall of the land of the machines; Neo meets his maker, and Trinity brings him back to life. With Aragorn and Arwen from *The Lord of the Rings* we witness Arwen surrendering her immortality to be with Aragorn. Together they witness the fall of Mordor, and Aragorn becomes the greatest king the world has ever known. They rule Middle Earth, and their reign is often referred to as the time of the golden years.

Finally we'll look at the example of Leonidas and Gorgo from the film *300,* based on the historical Battle of Thermopylae between the Spartan warriors and Persians in 480 BCE. King Leonidas of Sparta possesses the greatest strength ever known to man and becomes immortal, even through death, by victory. All of which he states would never have been possible without Queen Gorgo at his side. In this story we see a king and queen ruling side by side in equality for the very first time in ancient Greek culture. And no real surprise here: Sparta was the most abundant and powerful empire Greece had ever known. To this day the Spartan army commands huge recognition for the role it played in classical Greek culture.

Through this research I have come to realize that there is, in fact, *only one story* that keeps repeating itself on Earth. Whether it's written in our history books, religious texts, magical rituals, or personified in epic movies, it is the story of longing to joyfully merge with our twin soul while still here in the body. Is this the work of Sophia and the Logos? Is this El and Asherah playing out their divine plan of reuniting in human form?

There is only one way to find out, and that is to experience it for ourselves. Fortunately, we cannot read about this and expect to have the answers. The mystery of this subject becomes woven inside you as you come together in the fullness of this process.

Understanding and experiencing sacred union is critical to our world on both a micro- and macrolevel. In all the examples that exist there is always a building of tension, unrest, and disharmony upon the planet right before the twin souls unite. The birth of their union allows all that was corrupt to be destroyed and new civilizations to be formed. Nothing of ignorance could bear to stand in the light of their love.

Our time on Earth is nearing a similar upheaval. We, as a species, are being invited, or rather *urged,* to enter into sacred union on a massive level.

Because you *are* ready, you are invited to this temple of love. Because you are initiates, you are masters, you are teachers, you are healers, and you are lovers. And it is this embrace that must surround the world now. It is the embrace of the beloved. Know that this love is the eternal key, and I stand before you and with you on this path. You are worthy; you are the immaculate divine souls of light that *know* this. Go forth in faith. God's holy purpose serves through you, and there is only the path and only the way. And you show the way for your own soul, your spirit, your mind, your heart.

This is the epiphany. There is but one purpose for the truth: It is to be lived. And the world shall be revealed through this truth, through your living body, through surrender to sacred union.

It is not, however, merely one couple that will save the world this time—it must be many.

My question is, will it be you and your beloved?

I move forward with trust and consciousness.

PREPARATION
In the Beginning

Every soul ever created was forged in the Fires of Creation as "two in one." A soul made of one part male and one part female. These souls were left to cool intertwined around one another before the evitable separation that prepared them for their journey of reunion. Only in separation could they experience the fullness of their great and holy love. A love that would bring them back together with such a thunderous force that God wept in prostration.

ANAIYA SOPHIA,
PILGRIMAGE OF LOVE

Welcome to the world I live in. These words first came to me as I began to read *Pistis Sophia,* known as the Gnostic Bible, which was found underground in Egypt in 1773 and originally written in Coptic. You are embarking on a journey that intends to radicalize your mind, open your heart, and profoundly inspire you to live by your soul. This book is a mistress-piece of wild living, untameable existence, and a hallmark of the bravest hearts.

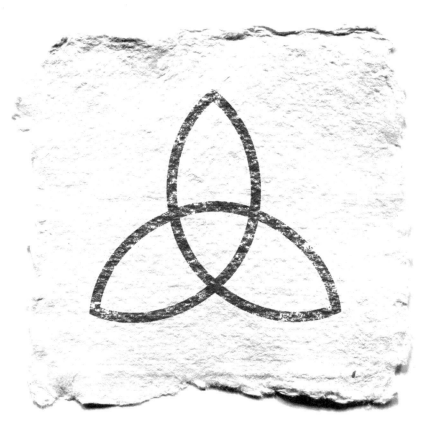

Threefold Flame

What you are about to read is based on a gnostic transmission. The word *gnostic* means "to know" or "knowledge." Allow yourself to read the words that follow without actually thinking or forming an opinion; simply relax into the experience of receiving this beautiful story. Tune your awareness to any sensations in the body, especially those that carry an emotional response. Whatever emotions and sensations arise, they are to be welcomed and given the space to be acknowledged and felt. If this writing resonates with you, I encourage you to record your own voice reading it. I have found that listening to this story in the warmth of one's bed, in the dim light, is the key to a doorway that unlocks very deep aspects within the soul.

The Original Separation

Once upon a time, while the universe was still cooling from the fires of creation, a clamoring cry resounded throughout the heavens, telling of a great darkness that had descended onto Earth.

Out of the heavens came she, the Holy Sophia, the Mother of all creation. Forsaking her divinity, she fell to Earth in a brave attempt to save her children. Awaiting her was a growing abomination: a powerful dark lord attempting to enslave the world by tormenting and separating human souls from her love.

In her last desperate act, consumed by the fierce compassion of her love, she fragmented into billions of little pieces, casting a spark of herself into every single one of her children. With her last breath, she cried out an almighty prayer, knowing that one day her redeemer would find her.

— ♦ —

And find her he does—inside each and every single one of us.

The story of Sophia is the story of our own soul and our longing for the love of our Creator. Like our own journey, the ascent is a slow and winding process full of initiations and adventures along the way. Yet one thing is certain—*amor vincit omnia* (love conquers all).

The victorious and ecstatic reunion of Sophia and her beloved Logos is *the* epic love story of all time, one that deep down we all wish to live.

One of the values of this story is the portrayal of the Logos as a hero figure, liberator, and lover. The savior comes to Sophia as the hero to rescue the damsel in distress, yet he does not pick her up and carry her back to the heavens; he gives her light power to rise above the chaos, to become more conscious of who she is in her own power. Her response is gratefulness, greater faith in the light and love. Like

Sophia, all our souls are damsels in distress, suffering the distress of the soul not knowing who she is and, like Sophia, besieged by mate rial powers. Until our response to receiving that light is an increase in gratefulness, faithfulness, and love, the liberator and lover is not revealed to us.

In their ecstatic reunion a fountain of light sparks, pours forth between them, and showers the world with its redemptive seed to empower all of the exiled light of Sophia that was placed in the souls of humankind to awaken and remember. In their powerful reunion they carve open the path for all souls to be able to enter sacred union and return home.

As above, so below . . .

And so, the alchemical initiation known as sacred union was birthed. It is the process that restores and reunifies twin souls on Earth so that the Logos can enter into the aspect of Sophia that is buried deep within us, holding the magnetics that attract us to the other half of our soul.

For now, that is where *this* story ends . . .

But here in this book is where we pick up the continuation of that story again. Within these pages, you will find the love, power, and wisdom that are needed to pull ourselves back together—literally. This is no New Age, wet-behind-the-ears, no-handle-on-reality, guru-led spiritual path. No, this is written from the very scream of life itself. Very few of us are willing to go on this journey for real, to use everything we've got to liberate ourselves, our partners, and the world into the deepest possible truth, love, and openness. Few men are willing to give their deepest genius, their true endowment, the poetry of their very being, with every thrust of their penetration into life. Most men are limp with doubt and uncertainty, whereas many women hold back from initiation quietly withholding because of their fear of being wounded, fear of being rejected. How on Earth did woman ever forget that the feminine principle is the very mistress of these earthly realms? Woman contains within her womb the power to initiate change in the real world and the ability to catalyze the situation to transform.

> We are all wounded, even the gurus and spiritual leaders of this world. Together we hold back our true drive because of fear. So instead, we diddle our partners and the world just enough to extract the pleasure and comfort we need to assuage our nagging sense of falsity and incompleteness. But if you are willing to discover and embrace your truth, lean through your fears, and give everything you've got, you can penetrate the world and your woman/man from the core of your being and bloom them into love without limit. You can ravish your woman so deeply that her surrender breaks your heart into light. You can press yourself into the world and your man with such enduring love that the world opens and receives your deepest gifts.
>
> David Deida,
> "Do It for Love"

Welcome to the world we currently live in. It's going to take work, and we have to become real. This journey is one of light and dark; in fact, it's more a journey of every spectral shade imaginable. Nothing is forbidden, nothing is denied, nothing is frowned upon; there is only one rule, and that is:

Love one another.

Let's take a breather. . . .

Ready to continue?

First of all, when I speak of the masculine and feminine, I am not speaking about men and women. We all carry within us both the masculine and feminine principles. One of our most important contributions to this path is to first create a sacred union within, a harmonious blend of our own internal masculine and feminine energies.

Second, I openheartedly believe that twin souls take form as both opposite and same sex gender. I do not hold the energy that twin souls can only be a male/female dynamic. However, with same-sex couplings, there will still need to be an obvious and integrated balance of masculine and feminine energies within both people.

Now that we have got those issues out of the way, let's continue.

Below are the definitions for soul mate and twin soul so that you can better understand for yourself this process and navigate where you are in terms of your current relationships.

TWIN SOULS

Twin souls are forged from the fires of creation at the very same time and left to cool entwined around each other. Created without individualized gender, they rest inside one another for eons until there is an inner movement that causes them to separate and cast themselves in opposite directions from each other. Their destiny is to receive the knowledge of polar opposite experiences so that when they eventually reunite, they create a richer, more varied tapestry that inevitably weaves them back together.

The incessant throbbing of desire and longing for the other twin is never far beneath the subconscious. It becomes more and more coherent as the soul evolves in terms of his or her actualization. Before the reunification process some of the initiations created to bring them closer are often fraught with suffering, as the ego dissolves, making way for the soul. That means that even though we meet our twin, it may not be a blissful reunion for us. Pain and suffering can beset the twins, as they carry within them the memories and pain of their long journey to finally find each other again. When they do eventually meet, there is an inner dragon they have to slay together—and that is the fear of losing one another. These feelings and emotions are colossal in twin souls and have to be dealt with as gently as possible *before* entering into sacred union.

However, one of the main differences is that their love for one another is always steadfast and enduring. They consistently love and long for one another, because their love is eternal and continues far beyond their human experiences. Like two oppositely oriented magnets they are constantly pulled back together, receiving medicine and healing the moment they connect.

They reunite when one or both of them have worked through enough of their intergender emotional wounds so that the light of the soul can begin to attract and draw the other half toward itself. When they meet they are invited by their souls to harness the power of their love and merge to continue on as one for the rest of their journey until they reach the fullness of love. It is only at this stage of the journey, when they meet and commit to the merging, that they can go deeper into their soul progression. Between them there is no experience that has not been lived through. Those in the presence of reunified twin souls find that all their questions end as all answers are found—not because reunified souls are special or blessed but because the very nature, the unified energies, of two souls merged as one can heal and transform. They offer a completed space where others can find sanctuary resting within their love and consciousness.

Those who live spiritual lives of emotional detachment often do so when they are unable or unwilling to face their twin soul. For many being in love is not a sign of spiritual intelligence—quite the opposite. It can be an overwhelming, life-altering experience to come face-to-face with the other half of your soul. Many people flee in emotional terror and allow emotional baggage to destroy the process. But when they accept this beautiful opportunity, it can and will become the most intensely transformative and powerful experience of their lives. Whatever the case, there is no force on Earth that can keep twin souls apart, but human choices can absolutely delay their reunion.

When meeting a twin soul we may have some preconceived romantic notions about who and what he or she is and will be for us. We conjure up great expectations about this love and how it will turn out. The ironic thing about expectations is that while some of them are met, some may be cruelly dashed and others will far surpass our original expectations.

Let the beloved do its work with and for you. Stay conscious, communicate, and consummate as often as possible. Within the remembrance of your union, all worldly affairs diminish. In my opinion the yin-yang symbol is a perfect representation of the original soul template, made up of both masculine and feminine principles.

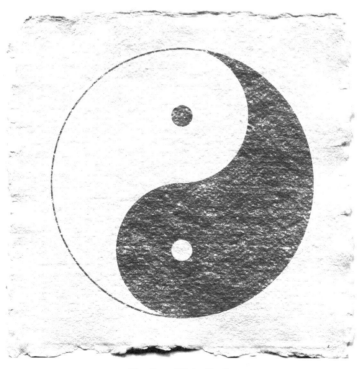

Yin-Yang/Twin Soul

Hallmarks of a Twin Soul

Immediate recognition hits as a barrage of feelings and sensations of intense magnetism and longing. Even the sound of his or her name will confirm the identity of the twin soul. There really is no need to go to clairvoyants or psychics to find out who your twin soul is. No one knows, apart from you, and the moment you come into one another's consciousness, you shall know with every fiber of your being. Whether you meet face-to-face, or you hear about him or her through friends, online, or in passing, you will know and will have no doubt.

After the initial coming together there will be some intense challenges to overcome. Remember, you have both experienced many kinds of polar opposite understandings. Every type of duality (pairs of opposites) may arise to be played out until there is nothing left but love and an incredible desire to merge and become one. Also, we have to recognize that every intergender wound that we may be carrying has to be transformed. Every hurt, betrayal, fear, and distrust of the opposite gender (or same sex) has to be healed. You may think that you have healed this, but it will only be in relating to your twin soul that the most painful aspects arise.

One of the classic hallmarks that you have found your twin soul is that the idea of being two becomes completely repellent. Twin souls yearn constantly to merge into one. It is their natural state. There is also a heightened sensitivity; you will be able to feel one another's emotional responses, even if it is denied, because your twin is you, and you are your twin. You are the one soul.

This is why it is imperative that there is a period of preparation before you enter the sacred union process.

SOUL MATES

Soul mates are souls created close to you at the time of the original creation. I often refer to the Flower of Life sacred geometry as a visual

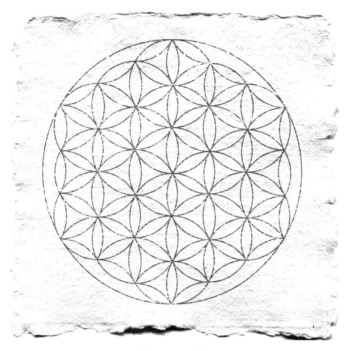

Flower of Life

example of the cluster formation in which human souls may have been originally formed. The Flower of Life has six associated circles (souls) linked around a seventh circle (twin soul). Drawing from my personal journey of research and experience, I sense that we each have twelve soul mates, quite possibly six female and six male. Each of these twelve soul halves will carry the energetic signature of the twelve houses of the zodiac and their twelve associated planets. However, from the illustration you will see that there are another six soul clusters forming within the original. These other clusters are all connected and interwoven within the soul matrix. Therefore, in total there are 144 souls making up one soul family.

The purpose of meeting and engaging with a soul mate is to create a two-way relationship that refines, sculpts, and shapes the other individual into becoming more of him- or herself. Soul mates bring out the qualities and strengths within each soul as a way of preparing one another for when the time and space is right for the twin soul reunion.

The way this happens is that soul mates continually present a mirror to us so we may peel away distortions to find our inner completeness. Through this process we are refining constantly into the full expression of our individuality. Looking in the mirror is not always something we may wish to do—especially if what we see doesn't agree with us! And to intensify matters, there is simply no escaping the mirror once it's shown to us, especially when it feels like all our buttons get pressed at once. With our soul mate we are continually exposed to the good, the bad, and the ugly!

For a soul that is just beginning on this Earth, this process would be too destructive, and so union with our soul mate doesn't usually happen at the same place or time until a soul has released sufficient suffering and let go of remaining emotional attachments along the path. Soul mates don't get to meet on Earth unless both are ready to move onto a higher plane of existence as part of their spiritual journey.

When soul mates unite there is no allowance for anything other than pure honesty and clarity between them. Distortions will surface immediately to be released. Frequently people go through many relationships that help to fine-tune and release attachments until they are sufficiently evolved to move on to higher paradigms with their soul mates. Of course we may often experience deeply fulfilling relationships with someone other than a soul mate before we get there. It is all part of the grand unfolding of the re-creation of the unique soul.

When you meet a soul mate there is also an instant recognition, a familiarity that brings with it a wondrous joy and feeling of belonging. Soul mates are in each other's lives to offer support, love, and kindness. There is a timeless feeling when soul mates are together. In fact, they'll often find themselves saying, "It feels like I've known you forever." All soul mate relationships are for the purpose of spiritual growth and the deepening and expanding of all spiritual attributes. Soul mates teach each other how to love themselves and then how to love each other, thereby creating the most ideal situation for a conscious family.

Not all soul mate reunions are sexual; many of them will be purely platonic, based on friendship, collaboration, and deep spiritual support. Soul mates will literally serve one another for years as they both learn and experience how to embody unconditional love.

Hallmarks of a Soul Mate

A warm and comfortable feeling when together. Feelings of support, friendship, family, and familiarity. A strong attraction. You may adore and love the way the other person looks, enjoying his or her entire being. But you will always be two individuals, using your time together to strengthen and develop your separate identities. No desire to merge; happy and content to enjoy individuality and two-ness.

HOW TO APPROACH THIS JOURNEY

There will most likely be three categories of individuals reading this book.

* Single people
* People in a newly formed relationship
* People in a long-term relationship

Let me first speak to the people in a relationship. If you desire to go on this journey and you *know* that the person you are in relationship with is not a soul mate or your twin soul—end the relationship.

It's really that simple. For those who feel they are in a relationship with their soul mate, this process will still continue to attract the twin soul. As you progress along this path you will either realize, once your wounds have been healed, that your soul mate is in fact your twin soul, or you will speed up the duration of your time with your soul mate and reach a place of completion within the relationship. Either way the space for the twin soul opens up.

If you continue to deny what you already know and stay in a

relationship that is not taking you into the depths, you will not only be holding yourself back from progressing in love and life, but the other person will be held back as well, for love that is not requited in equal measure is not love at all, is not sacred. And holding on to the ideal of such love can keep us from finding the one that is true.

We all truly have to begin this journey from a clear and clean slate.

As for the single readers, in some respects you are in a great place as you can use this book as a way to prepare deeply on every level and attract your beloved toward you.

Where to Begin

Please pay close attention to this wisdom. This is a very powerful initiation containing the fullness of your existence and the many dimensional layers of your being. One has to respect and acknowledge the enormity of the task at hand. We cannot push past the natural rhythm and flows of this journey. I tried and got burned many times. Only in hindsight can I report back to you with the advice to move slowly and thoroughly. I have been working with the template of a nine-month gestation process based entirely on the three trimesters of human pregnancy. By breaking the threefold flame into three, three-month preparatory periods, we arrive at nine months. The last month (thirty days) is given to the sacred union ritualistic ceremony, which brings us to ten months in total. As we will come to discover, ten is the number of spheres in the Tree of Life, the esoteric map of how we came from the godhead into manifestation and how we can reverse the journey.

So now we stand at the threshold of the most important part of this journey—the preparation stage. The majority of this book will cover this preparatory aspect in a very complete way. We will cover the three main areas of sacred union based on the threefold flame of gnostic Christianity (power, love, and wisdom) as well as the Holy Trinity in all forms of alchemy (feminine, God, and masculine), as well as the law of three found within science and nature (negative, neutral, and positive).

It breaks down like this:

* Sexual sacredness: power, feminine, negative (first trimester)
* Emotional intimacy: love, God, neutral (second trimester)
* Soul consciousness: wisdom, masculine, positive (third trimester)

It is at this point that we begin to sincerely open to God, the third element. It is not possible to do this work without the Creator of our soul, as it is the soul that is drawing us together and it is the soul where we continue after death. Sacred union does not end when we die, and it is not limited to sacred sexuality as often misrepresented in the New Age arena. In order to reach the full potential of this work we have to heal all and every wound that we may carry regarding God our Creator, as we will be relying heavily upon his/her love and truth to progress. When we look at the alchemical image of the caduceus, which is also symbolic of Mercury and means higher forms of communication, we see a figure of two serpents wrapped around a center rod. The rod is a symbol

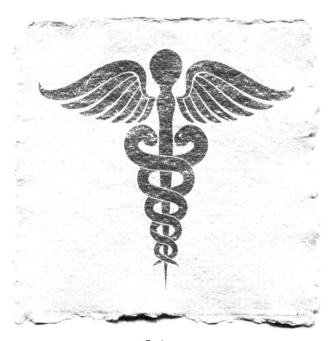

Caduceus

of the transforming alchemical power (love/God). The two serpents represent polarity or duality (power/feminine and wisdom/masculine). By alchemizing all three elements together, we discover the alchemical meaning of balance, duality, and unity.

My suggestion is for you to take nine months in total to prepare. On the tenth month you enter the process of sacred union. To ignore or overlook this advice would be a huge mistake. I have walked this path, I have studied this path, and I live and breathe this path. Please do not rush in to the final phase without preparing.

These three aspects are the most powerful centers of our being, and it will be these three streams of energy that will merge in the sacred union process. The basics of sacred union work a lot like a three-pinned electrical plug. It's where you will plug into one another, and from there a multitude of endless subtle and refined delicacies of energetic fusion shall unfold (more on that soon!).

After we take an in-depth look at the preparation process we will explore the sacred union process. Another word of caution: even if you did attempt to enter into the process of sacred union with a partner who was not your twin soul (soul half), you would not be allowed to fulfill the process. In my personal journey I have twice made the error of trying to enter sacred union with a soul mate, and both times life powerfully intervened and brought the process to an abrupt end. There are guardians to this work, and they will not allow souls to join who are not destined to. Bear in mind, of course, that once you have moved through the preparatory stages there will be no doubt as to who is or isn't your twin soul.

Within each part of the three sections you will find theory, practice for yourself, and practice to share with your partner. If you do not have a partner you can work with your twin soul in the energetic realms, until he or she manifests in the physical world.

This process will move thoroughly throughout your entire system as depicted with the pentagram (see p. 30). Its meaning is quite the opposite of its unfortunate reputation, the pentagram (pentacle) is a symbol

Pentagram of our existence

of harmony, health, and mystic powers. The Pythagoreans adopted it as a sign of health and the sacred marriage of heaven and Earth. As a symbol of heaven and Earth, as well as a symbol for human being, the pentagram holds great power—so much so that it was used as a protective emblem among alchemists and magicians alike. Specifically, alchemists would press this symbol on hermetic books to emphasize the knowledge within as being protected and sacred. The pentagram is also the symbol for Venus. That is why when carving open the path of sacred union I knew to include the whole of our existence in the exercises and processes that will prepare us in the following five areas.

* Physical
* Sexual
* Emotional
* Mental
* Soulful

By following this route I assure you that you will become primed and ready to either manifest your twin soul or enter into sacred union. The process you are about to move through is based on what is known as layered learning, a method once used in the ancient mystery schools. This means that as you learn in a cognitive way (reading the words and forming understanding) there will be another process happening alongside your awareness that will begin to unfold during your dream time. Deeper insights will be formed through your dreams and altered states. This is a gnostic process that you are entering. And that means that only 10 percent of the process can be learned in a traditional sense. The rest will be given to you through mystical initiation.

At the end of every chapter there will be a sacred initiation. This is a conscious step that is taken along the path of preparing for sacred union. This section will contain a mystical step to take for those walking this path as a single woman (handmaiden) or single man (light bearer) and those entering into sacred union with a partner. Like a true alchemist I have broken down everything into its intrinsic steps and stages. Follow this path and you will be consciously aligning with the natural rhythms and flow of the creative forces in the universe. As we learn to balance knowledge with the surrender to the mystery, it is advisable to carefully follow these steps. You will know when you hear the voice and sense the presence of the mystery. In that moment there are no more doubts. You simply *know*.

The last piece of sacred advice is to choose the *moment* you begin to take this journey. Powerful dates are an excellent place to start—such as new moons, equinoxes, solstices, mirror dates (12-12-12), or your birthday. Perhaps you have your own knowing of when to start. Whatever it is, make the whole process a ritual: buy a new journal to record the experience, and make the commitment to yourself and your twin soul to live and breathe this process.

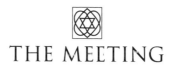

THE MEETING

The meeting is one of the most powerful moments on this path. You may *think* you have no control over when you meet and that this destined moment is held in the hands of fate—I do not believe that to be so. You decide the moment you will meet in the mystery by calling forth the presence of your twin soul in meditation or deep relaxation, but what you do with that moment is what truly counts. In the Sufi tradition there is a mystery that is known as nazar, which means "the glance" or gift. Rumi and Shams often spoke about how a spiritual alchemy takes place inside the glance. It is as if the meeting happens inside the two of you. If you have a chance to discuss this in person when you eventually meet, you will discover this truth. Within the eyes of your soul family, there is an electrical charge transmitted and received. Those united in a soul family cannot *not* know that it has happened. As for twin souls, the charge is intensified. The question is, are you willing enough to stay present and open to receive such a glance?

The meeting first happens in the ethers.

Sacred Initiation

If you are single and you haven't already called forth this sacred initiation, do so when you feel the right time and space. If you are not single, consciously tune in to your partner energetically to open a dialogue with the intention to bring forth the physical meeting of twin souls. Declare powerfully that you are ready to meet, as you scan and scope for any fears or uncertainties that may arise, and then attend to them consciously, feeling every emotion and sensation and owning them.

Recognizing the Physicality and Energy of the Meeting

1. First things first: When you meet you will know it. You may deny it, but secretly to yourself, in the middle of the night, you will know. When it happens, pay attention. Be open to offer and receive the glance. There will be a moment when the window of opportunity opens for the glance to happen.

   When all of your heart is in your body and one meets a beloved, the meeting is immediate, direct, and real. When your pure woman-ness is in all your body, you know him, you see him, you find him, you reach him, you love him. And of course, the same for the men.

2. Women—you are invited to let the other in. Allow yourself the per-mission to receive the glance from your beloved. Begin to gently tune in to his energy, the rhythm, the depth, the flow and temperature. Be aware of his energy gently coming in to your body awareness and configuration.

3. Men—you are invited to gently push your energy forward and wait until you receive her permission. When it is given (acknowledged through feeling and sensing), respectfully penetrate her energy field, feeling her internal energetic fields and flows. Become aware of the two in one.

I move forward with trust and consciousness.

PART ONE

Sacred Sexuality

The First Trimester

Make me, O Lord, nourishment for the blazing flame. . . .
Make me, O God, food for the sacred fire.

KAHLIL GIBRAN,
"AT THE DOOR OF THE TEMPLE"

1
ENTERING
THE ALCHEMICAL
MARRIAGE

Back in the days of legend and lore, there are stories of how there has always been an ancient lineage that carried the sacred and royal bloodline of kings and queens, not of an earthly kingdom but more of a spiritual domain. We are told that this soul family has been on Earth since the beginning of time and that the original carriers of the flame were Adam and Eve. In my opinion this ancestral lineage has nothing to do with blood and is not a set of traits and genes that are passed on to offspring. This bloodline is more of a soul longing that gets ignited by the mystery itself, to know thyself. This longing is a profoundly soulful emotional energy that is held and activated throughout the soul and subtle anatomy (light bodies) as mapped out by the Tree of Life. There are also three atomic forces—positive, negative, and neutral—held within the sacral, heart, and third eye chakras that carry the fullness of the flame. This flame is the *ruach,* the life force, the vital spark, the juice and magic evident in those who follow the longing. The absolute truth is that everyone carries the flame inside them, but a carrier of the flame is one who knows and lives this. I am writing this book for you, the carriers of the flame reading this, because sacred union is an essential part of this legendary legacy. We know that it was through separation that we "fell" to Earth and that to return means reunion.

It is by love (trust/feminine) and light (consciousness/masculine) that we return. Love is revealed through the feminine principle as touch, relaxation, being, playfulness, healing, creation, passion, compassion, ecstasy, expression through words, art, bodily movement, enjoyment, and all aspects of relationship. Light is revealed through the masculine principle as truth, knowledge, stillness, navigation, direction, choice, clarity, and actions taken in the outer world.

CARRIERS OF THE FLAME

Pioneers, visionaries, nonconformists, innovators, revolutionaries, mystics, poets, artists, bearers of the truth, way seers—those who fearlessly express the spirit and juice of life by giving form to the Holy Spirit and the celebration of freely being alive. Those who are free to create and free to destroy.

Some qualities of a carrier of the flame are endless enthusiasm, the outpouring of love, spiritual fire, soulful insight, passion, devotion, genius, beauty, grace, and excitement. These creative, gloriously inspired souls are absolutely hardwired to change the world. They are here to comfort the disturbed and to disturb the comfortable!

There must always be carriers of the flame on Earth as it is their purpose to shed light and shower love on the madness of society—to continually resurrect the timeless transcendent spirit of truth. Their mission is to bring truth through the revelation of God's love and its inherent power during the darkest of times. Within this family of light, there is the alchemical number of three paths of destiny: one for handmaidens, one for light bearers, and one for those who together enter into sacred union.

The Three Paths of Destiny

Handmaidens

These are women (and feminine men) who work alone to heal the sexually suppressed and brokenhearted as well as being the midwives of conscious birthing. Their purpose is to heal and love one another. Their essence of love is passed through waves of transmission during healing, teaching, dancing, speaking, singing, and lovemaking. Handmaidens use their sexual and emotional energies to heal and transform both men and women in an authentic and pure way. Their beloved is God, and through each one whom they serve, they serve God in the fullness. When a handmaiden serves a woman, she is serving Sophia the Divine Feminine. This is *not* a form of Tantra or sex magic. A handmaiden is a vessel of love. By any means necessary, she shall deliver that man or woman to the lap of God, taking him or her to the heights and depths, way beyond the everyday human experience into the realms of cosmic consciousness. How does she do that? Because she is "in love" with God, and she longs to serve the Divine with every fiber of her being. Her relationship with God is whole, integrated, and incredibly personal. She knows deeply that the fullness of God is both masculine and feminine and that both aspects desire to merge on Earth. She is fully aware of the rites of sacred union and may choose to enter that path with her twin flame. However, she is here on Earth to carve open the way and prepare all those who are destined for this journey.

The handmaiden's task is also to work intimately with the light bearers to "take the war out of them" by gently easing out any negative, dark, unconscious elements that need transforming. When light bearers focus all their masculine energy into either a high-frequency project using pure mental energy or an act of physical or energetic destruction, then it is only a handmaiden who can balance them out. She will know how to transmute the excessive masculine polarization into a harmonious balance by drawing them back into their bodies, through waves of pleasure and harmonization.

Light Bearers

These are men (and masculine women) who work alone to bring the light of God. They serve justice and truth, and they are the change makers whose task it is to pull down the old paradigm and craft and create the structures for the new one. They work with others by dragging them out of old paradigm thinking as they carve the way for a more creative expression of life to flow through them. They are pioneers of truth, way showers who are fearlessly unafraid of any form of resistance that holds old rules and programs in place. They deny nothing and will see to it that you do the same. They are free from fear within their own minds and know how the laws of justice work through them as well as the universal laws of our Creator and the cosmos that we live in.

These men are high-frequency holders of exceptional light and clarity, true innovators of our species. However, they will need to know a handmaiden to help them return to the harmonious balance of Earth by merging with her. This cooperation works both ways. A handmaiden experiences tremendous restabilization by being closely connected with a light bearer. Her wild shakti energy reconfigures into a more vertical pillar of light in the presence of a light bearer. This greatly assists her in grounding and anchoring herself and bringing her into a deep, silent, and still presence. Light bearers and handmaidens receive huge amounts of support and balance when they spend time in one another's presence. Any form of connection between them has beneficial results. In short, they need to work together by serving one another; this in turn restores the balance of the flame within them. Every handmaiden and light bearer needs to know and have regular contact with one another.

Sacred Union

These are light bearers and handmaidens who have recognized that they share the same soul essence and are ready and deeply desiring to reunify. Sacred union is the path for all twin souls who fully desire to reunite into their original creation template. When we look at the symbolic story of the Garden of Eden we see that it is by the act of separation that human beings "fell" to Earth. However, in a beautiful paradox, the way back to the Garden of Eden is through the gateway of reunion. When entering into sacred union through the restoration of the One Soul, the path of reunion is a highly charged and sacred act of returning to divinity. Instead of two people involved in the union, there are three: man, woman, and divinity. So again we see the sacred three, the work of the Holy Trinity: positive, negative, and neutral; mother, father, and Holy Spirit. The Holy Spirit is the ruach, the breath and fiery serpent of sexual energy, which powerfully, magnetically draws us together in longing and devotion. Within the ruach is the infinite energy for the "urge to merge" as contained within the story of the Logos and Sophia. Those who enter into this initiation will give their entire existence to the great work. The holy power that is unleashed through the reunion of the souls is immeasurable.

It is here where even the desire to work with others as a handmaiden or light bearer falls away. You enter into another world and dimension as you simply merge and become the flame itself. What happens during the great work, and what unfolds as a result of entering into it, truly belongs to the mystery. This is a deeply intimate and mystical experience and will no doubt have different meanings and expressions for everyone. I can offer you here the help and support you both may need for the path of sacred union—tools to clear the way from a human perspective and to take you through a process where all fears can be eradicated. There are ways and means to truly amp up the voltage within the holy sacred powers of the body, and these I will share with you as well.

Only a handmaiden and light bearer, and only those who are twin souls, can enter into sacred union, as their passionate sexual energy is one of the three keys that unlocks the door. The second key is love, fathomless love, devotion, and rapture. While the third key is the soulful longing for atonement with God (which *is* the sacred union state), only twin souls can unlock these energies. It begins the moment they lay eyes on one another. This divine mystery has been lost and perverted for too long. For countless centuries mystics and occultists have been using only the power of sexuality. This process has not worked, and in some cases it resulted in a tremendous distortion of intention. Only by the power of love can sacred union unlock its majestic gates and bring forth the full experience of holy matrimony of Sophia and the Logos in the reunification of the one soul.

Are You a Carrier of the Flame?

The question I always get asked is: "How do I know if I am a carrier of the flame?" Well, you *know* by feeling it deeply inside. You don't really have to ask the question. All carriers of the flame are born with a longing and desire within them that cannot and will not settle for the mundane and ordinary. There is something alive within them that can never rest until it discovers its source. They know in their hearts that there's a natural order to life, something more sovereign than any man-made rules or laws could ever express. They sense deep within themselves the pulse of life as the eternal substrate of the cosmos, as that which guides the very current of time and space. The innermost nature of their being comes alive with inspiration, passion, wisdom, enthusiasm, intuition, and spiritual fire—which are all aspects of love. They consistently sense the boundless order of existence and joyfully surrender to its will. When this is experienced by the mind, it is genius; when perceived through the eyes, it is beauty; when felt with the senses, it is grace; and when poured into the heart, it is an unspeakable expansion of love.

The flame is the mystery that cannot be seen yet is immensely felt and experienced. We all carry the flame, but only a handful of us have the capacity to recognize our ability and remember.

You will know immediately whether you were born to recognize your ability to be a carrier of the flame. I smile as I write this, because we simply know—but just in case you have momentarily forgotten:

* You burn with the desire to love God with every fiber of your existence.

* You ache with an intense longing to be dissolved and consciously enraptured by love.

* You are never satisfied with human love; you *know* there is more, much more.

* Your soul carries powerful and clear memories of being originally created in two (one masculine and one feminine), and you *know* you will meet your other half very soon if you've not already discovered him or her.

* You have felt the love of God and your beloved your whole life, and your desire to reunite with both is eternal.

* You have one foot in this world and another in the soulful realms

* You are moved by powerful emotions when you come in contact with Jesus Christ and Mary Magdalene, Isis and Osiris, and other beloved couples.

* You are touched by both the glory and downfall of ancient Egypt, the abuse of power in Atlantis, and the separation of masculine and feminine within Lemuria (these stories can be found on my *Wounds of Love* album).

* You burn with desire to be used as a vessel of love (feminine) and a messenger of light (masculine).

* Finally, you have a core commitment to remain humble and innocent in the continuous unfolding, ever hungry for God's love and the deepening of the mystery.

NASHAKH: THE KISS

The word *nashakh* is an ancient Hebrew word found in the Old Testament that means "to kiss with the soul." The deeper understanding of nashakh can be clearly tasted in the "Song of Songs" as written by King Solomon to his beloved Queen of Sheba. Here in this context we see that it means so much more than to kiss. In the "Song of Songs" we tantalizingly glimpse the potential that is laced within this divine kiss, known as the harmonious breath of the kiss, by consciously bringing our soul in to the alchemical chamber within our mouths. By breathing our souls on the lips of our beloved we give birth to one another through the sharing of the love that is within us, blending God with the self.

Through the sanctity of the kiss two souls come together to merge as one. This moment is a prelude to the sacred union of beloveds. When you receive and give this kiss there will be no doubting the enormity of what has just taken place. This is not simply a kiss but a meeting of souls, divinity, and the great mystery.

> When you drink from my mouth you will become like me, I myself shall become you, and the hidden things will be revealed to you.
> JESUS'S WORDS,
> FROM "RITUAL OF THE BRIDAL CHAMBER,"
> BY BISHOP ROSAMONDE MILLER

I feel that the "Song of Songs" is a map and esoteric recipe that contains the wisdom and the way of sacred union. Shrouded in mystery, encoded with symbolism, only carriers of the flame will be able to read between the lines and shine light over its paradoxical parables. It is written in a language of the soul, one that the mind can never grasp. It stirs nostalgic memories as it touches the deep essence within, and if you have the eyes to see and ears to hear you will understand its transmission.

The song begins with a kiss for this is the most sacred form of expression between beloveds. This kiss, the nashakh, means to breathe in harmony in a way that combines the souls of two into one, to share the same breath, to blend the life forces in a single coming together. The body, in its great intelligence, hungers to fall into the same breathing rhythm as the beloved by passing breath to one another through the mouth, encapsulated within the kiss and touch of one another's tongues. Note that this is different from the form of pranayama within the yab-yum (Tibetan Buddhism) tradition where you consciously inhale one another's breath.

> You may conquer with the sword, but you are the one that is conquered by a kiss.
>
> DANIEL HEINSIUS (1580–1655)

The nashakh is timeless and spaceless and happens within the soul. It has nothing to do with practices and spiritual disciplines; it is free of all boundaries and structures. It is the kiss that is laced with our Creator's great love, spiked with devotion and gratitude. To surrender means to lose ourselves within the waves of our rapture that urge us to give and receive until we become *anthropos,* which is to say fully realized human beings. This is the true meaning of nashakh.

Through this kiss we are reborn. We give birth to one another through this kiss by sharing the love within us with full trust and consciousness and by inviting in the fullness of God's presence. We release all our ideas of being human as we throw open the doors of our soul presence and unbridled love for the One that created us. We become pure unbounded energy that kisses and undulates throughout the entire universe, creating stars and galaxies along the way!

When looking at this experience from an energetic perspective we can see that when two individuals merge there is the introduction of a third circle—God/Creator/Source—that creates a sacred geometry known as the *vesica piscis*. The vesica piscis is used in a wide range of symbolism and can be seen as:

* the joining of God and Goddess
* a symbol for Jesus Christ
* the vagina of the female goddess
* the basic motif in the Flower of Life
* an overlay of the Tree of Life
* a geometrical description of square roots and harmonic proportions

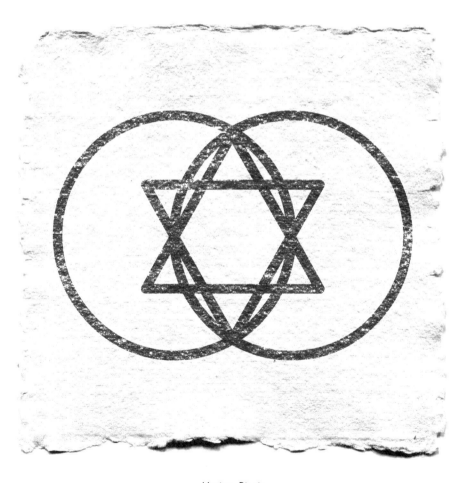

Vesica Piscis

The decision to kiss for the first time is the most crucial in any love story. It changes the relationship of two people in love far more strongly than even the final surrender because this kiss already has within it that surrender.

EMIL LUDWIG,
OF LIFE AND LOVE

When we receive this kiss there is a reawakening, rebirth, and reunion within the body. It is crucial that this first step be taken as this reawakening must happen within the body—for everything exists within the body and only by this awakening will we have the eyes to see and the ears to hear. Only through this awakening will you as a soul recognize and remember those with whom it is your destiny to reunite. You will know when you have received it—and you will also know when you have given it. If you feel the desire to give such a kiss yet hold back out of fear of losing yourself within the experience, be brave and take the leap of faith; have faith that life will expand until it fills the entire universe.

TIMING IS EVERYTHING: THE IMPORTANCE OF TIME AND SPACE

Everything happens according to time and space. You cannot stop or change time, but you can *alter* and *work with* space to improve your destiny.

According to the Kabbalah the most priceless wisdom is the knowledge contained within the laws of nature and the timings and rhythm of the cycles that govern us. We are told that the world was created and organized in a pattern of 3-7-12. These numbers correspond directly with the divine, astral, and physical worlds.

For our purposes here, in regard to the timing of the nashakh, we shall use the law of seven. Throughout the remainder of the book we shall endeavor to unfold the meaning of the other two numeric and dimensional realms, but first let us look at the number seven and the way it works in our lives.

Many things in the universe follow the rhythm of seven.

* Seven chakras
* Seven creative planets
* Seven wonders of the world
* Seven days of the week
* Seven seas
* Seven deadly sins
* Seven days of creation
* Seven archangels

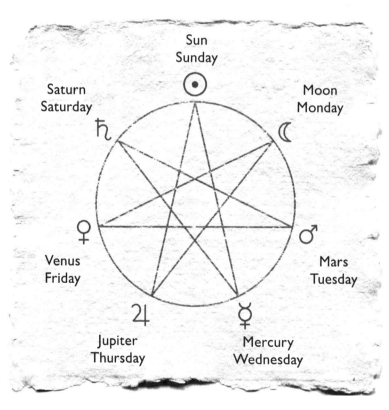

Seven Pointed Star, Planets, and Days

From the moment of your birth, the rhythm of seven began. Whichever day of the week you were born on, the vibration and frequency of that day's corresponding planet sculpts and influences your entire life. Learning to work with its attributes is essential to finding your purpose and fulfilling your destiny. Not only will you be working with the vibration of your planetary influence, you will also need to know the other greater rhythms of seven that are cycling around you constantly.

We are told in the Kabbalah that it was God that designed and created this sequence during the seven days of creation. On the first day he said, "Let there be light" (sun), and on the second day he said, "Let there be water" (moon). According to the Kabbalah, God was working with the seven great archangels who work through the seven creative planets to create Earth and all life upon it.

Now why am I telling you this? Because these seven planets are under the influence of the law of three—positive, negative, and neutral. This means that some planets have positive and life-enhancing qualities, some have negative heavy energies that, no matter what you do, you will never be able to fully overcome them, and others have a harmonious balance and neutralizing effect.

THE LAWS OF SEVEN AND THREE

Day of the Week	Planet and Energy	Charge
Sunday	Sun (good fortune)	Positive
Monday	Moon (visualizing and imagining intentions)	Neutral
Tuesday	Mars (physical energy)	Negative
Wednesday	Mercury (communication)	Neutral
Thursday	Jupiter (money matters and travel)	Positive
Friday	Venus (love and beauty)	Positive
Saturday	Saturn (rest and payment of debt)	Negative

What does this have to do with sacred union?

Everything.

The moment you meet, initiate the kiss, consummate the union, make a decision together, decide to marry, move in together, travel, or whatever; everything will be under the influence of the law of seven. I want you to be equipped with the knowledge of when to initiate according to the time and space that plays out on Earth. Backed by the favoritism of the planets or gods, according to Greek mythology, you will receive the push and grace of the universe, whereas making a false move will cause unnecessary hardships and added weight to the task at hand.

To truly understand this wisdom it is essential that you find out on which day of the week you were born and then on that day apply this sequence. For example, I was born on a Monday, so my personal week looks like this:

* Monday: Sun, positive
* Tuesday: Moon, neutral
* Wednesday: Mars, negative
* Thursday: Mercury, neutral
* Friday: Jupiter, positive
* Saturday: Venus, positive
* Sunday: Saturn, negative

Not only do we have to become aware of the rhythm of seven within our personal week, but we also have to become aware of a greater cycle of seven that maps out and unfolds within one of our Earth years. This greater cycle is made up of fifty-two seven-day cycles that mark our planetary periods over the course of the year, beginning and ending on our birthdays. For example, my birthday is on the December 22. That becomes the first day of my fifty-two-day sun period. After that I enter fifty-two days of my moon period and so on and so forth until I reach my Saturn period, roughly six weeks before my birthday, give or take a day or so depending on whether it's a leap year.

Therefore make sure you learn how the fifty-two-day periods unfold within your life and learn them by heart. It is *vital* that you initiate your intimacy with your beloved during the positive or neutral periods for both of you. Never ever do anything in your negative periods, or even if just one of you is in a negative period. Otherwise you will carry that negative imprint into your creations. My very best advice would be to initiate during Sun, Jupiter, and Venus periods and on a Sun, Jupiter, or Venus day.

Everything happens according to time and space. With this wisdom you will be able to navigate the forces at play and become a master at the game of life rather than a hapless victim. Knowledge is the key to success.

The Moon

Finally one last piece of knowledge that must never be overlooked is the timing of the moon. The moon, so intimately linked to Earth, not only influences the tides and the plant growth but also humanity's affairs as well. During the waxing phase, which is the new to full moon growing bigger in the sky each night, the lunar energies are at their most intense. During the waning phase the energies are dying down. The most powerful time to initiate anything is during the fourteen days of the waxing phase between the new and full moon. This time is the most propitious for productivity, growth, and abundance. Any project, venture, or coming together will naturally receive the full blessing of the moon to ensure the beautiful growth of all that becomes seeded during this phase.

It is worth noting that should you wish to remove unwanted things from your life, it is best to do this during the waning phase. For example, it is best to start a period of healing or to end a relationship when the moon is descending.

THE EGREGORE:
THE THIRD ELEMENT

The term *egregore* is derived from a Greek word meaning "to be aware of" or "to watch over." In magical esoteric circles an egregore is commonly understood to be a magical psychic entity consciously or unconsciously created by a couple or a group as an encapsulation and merger of their collective aspirations and ideals. The egregore appears to have been used as a source of psychic power—tapped in to together as a couple and for individual work as a source of fortitude and resolve. The egregore helps in the collective developmental aspirations of a couple or group.

The egregore is birthed the moment any bodily liquids merge or when any deep, prolonged, focused spiritual energy is raised together. Your egregore is the creation of a living and feeling being that has its own awareness and intelligence. It exists, it feels, and it longs for you to be together. When close relationships break down and there is a separation, it is the tearing apart of the egregore that causes the deep soulful pain of breaking up. The egregore, when created consciously, contains our innocence, trust, love, and endless magnetism to be together as one. It does not know the ways of human egoic thinking and being in this world. It knows only one thing—reunion. It is the total combination of your love and desire to be together. The egregore can be used to communicate telepathically with one another, to stay consciously linked even when physically apart, and also as a source of wise counsel to assist the full potential of your union. The egregore carries the reason why you came together and the fullness of your destiny.

Like any other being that may experience being torn apart, when there is a breakup in a relationship the egregore will flood the two people involved with hormonal responses that are loaded with memories and feelings designed to trigger them to consider getting back together. That is why it is important to not get involved with someone who is recently out of a relationship, as their old egregore will still be present and influencing their decisions and choices. This is also one of the greatest reasons why we have to work so hard on the inner planes when we separate from someone to clear us of this psychic entity and all the bonds and threads woven within us that link us to the other person.

When you create the egregore in a fresh and conscious way, you will find a bottomless wealth of wisdom and sanctuary within its knowledge. The egregore, when created in trust and consciousness, becomes the voice and space of the unified soul that has a timeless and eternal link with God. When you initiate with the nashakh and kiss with the breath and essence of your soul, the signature and frequency of the souls begin to conceive the building blocks of the egregore. This "immaculate conception" carries the virginal essence so that your egregore can be birthed in absolute purity and celestial love.

The problem we face as a species is that we have lost this ancient knowledge, yet we continue to create egregores in ignorance and lust. Instead of creating the third element in love we give birth instead to needy or controlling children—egregores that whine and cringe when there is separation or lack of attention. This kind of egregore will inevitably end up destroying a relationship due to its suffocating intoxication. This is often because the necessary qualities of consciousness were not present at its birth, and the knowledge of time and space was not known. Instead of the egregore being a creation of soul union it most likely is a result of unconscious agendas and conditions. Like everything in this life, you reap what you sow.

If you kiss with innocence, love, trust, and consciousness your egregore shall shine forth with those qualities. If you are full of lust, control, and an agenda then you shall give birth to that quality of being.

Thus we have the Holy Trinity: positive (masculine), negative (feminine), and neutral (egregore). Consciously used, these are the basic building blocks for true alchemy. The question becomes: Once you have birthed your third element what are you going to create together?

THE FIVE OFFERINGS

After you have kissed and you know deep inside that you wish to progress further, the next stage will be the initiation of the five offerings, which are based on the five senses. These five items will be left with your partner for a period of time until he or she has been accepted completely into the sensory awareness of the other. You can do this in person as well as energetically. Both partners are to give and receive the five offerings.

Sacred Initiation

You are being invited to offer five gifts that carry the energetic and sensory signature of your soul and not your personality.

1. An offering of a visual image of your soul (art, photo, image, color, film clip, illustration).
2. An offering of the sound of your soul (piece of music, soundscape, you singing, soundtrack from film)
3. An offering of the smell of your soul (drop some oil or perfume onto a handkerchief or piece of paper as you need to be able to leave the scent with him or her)
4. An offering of the taste of your soul in food or drink
5. An offering of the touch of your soul (fabric, crystal to handle, sacred object, some tangible item that the other can handle)

When you are not together your intention will be to keep the energy building and to weave together even at a distance. These sensory offerings from one soul to the other will help deepen the connection as you build toward the great work of sacred union.

I move forward with trust and consciousness.

2

THE ALCHEMY OF LOVE

Feeling dirty, ashamed, and damaged, she hid her story.
Not knowing that the woman next to her also hid hers.
And the next woman, and the next. Finally someone
whispered the truth. And their eyes met, and their tears
came, their heads nodded softly, and their arms reached
out. Holding each other gently, telling their stories, the
healing began.

TERRI ST. CLOUD, *HER WHITE TREE*

This section of the book takes us on a profound healing journey. All of us carry personal wounds found within our sexuality and our relationships with the opposite gender. As you read through this wisdom and progress through the clearings and corrections, first apply every step to your *own* individual process. If you are already in relationship, when it feels right you can begin this sacred sexuality journey *together* by moving and breathing as you travel through the seven gates while making love. It is important to take your time and slow everything down in order to consciously explore and feel each domain with the masculine and feminine principles on both the inner and outer levels.

WHAT ARE
THE SEVEN GATES?

For an in-depth understanding of the seven gates please refer to my book *Womb Wisdom: Awakening of the Creative and Forgotten Powers of the Feminine* (Destiny Books). You can also listen to my guided meditation through the seven gates on my CD *Womb*. In the meantime you will find a summary here.

I often refer to the first three gates in both men and women as being the internal landscape upon which our personal sexual story is encoded. All traumas and sexual wounds of a physical and energetic nature will be located in the first three gates, while I see the fourth gate as the bridge between worlds. For a woman the first gate is the cervix, a thin, long tunnel that leads to the entrance of the womb. For a man this gate is the lips of the lingam, the part of him that can "kiss" the cervix as he slowly docks in the energetic matrix that is opening another dimensional space before him.

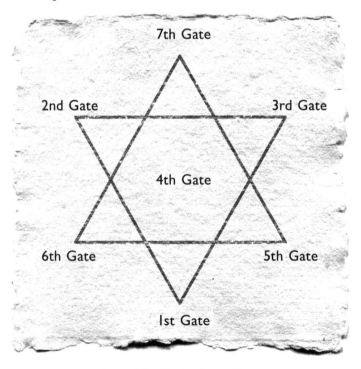

Star of David, the Seven Gates

THE SEVEN GATES

	First Gate	Second Gate	Third Gate	Fourth Gate	Fifth Gate	Sixth Gate	Seventh Gate
Element	Earth	Water	Fire	Air	Ether	None	None
Body Part (Feminine)	Labia	G-spot	Clitoris	Cervix	Entrance of the womb	Conception point in the womb	*Through the sixth gate into the void*
Body Part (Masculine)	Perineum	Prostate	Length of lingam	Lips of lingam	Entrance of the womb	Conception point in the womb	*Through the sixth gate into the void*
Associated Gland	Adrenal	Ovaries (fem.)/ Testes (masc.)	Pancreas	Thyroid or para-thyroid	Thymus	Pineal	Pituitary
Emotional Key	Trust	Gratitude	Devotion	Nonduality	Rapture	Grace	Surrender
Shadow Qualities	Fear, distrust, frigidness, impotence, disassociation, disconnection	Bitter, hard, spiteful, cruel, cold	Fiery, aggressive, angry, turbulent, explosive, projective	Jekyll and Hyde type of switching and disjointed personality, bi-polar, schizophrenic; manifests as Eve and Lilith in a woman and Christ and Pan in a man, forming a schism between the light and dark aspects of sexuality	Polarized in one principle (masculine or feminine), intergender wounds, distrust of masculine and feminine, ineffectual, lack of direction (too feminine), lack of creative manifestation (too masculine)	Egoic, self-centered, self-reliant, independent, self-interested, invested in material world and gain	Last remaining threads of resistance, the last holdout, deepest secret places, and areas unwilling to surrender to the godhead, the movement from "my will" to "thy will"
Luminescent Qualities	Feminine: accepting, inviting, open, warm, magnetic; Masculine: penetrative, fully present and consistent; Both: connected to the web of all life	Sweet, delicious, Divine nectar, playful, innocent	Feminine: exceptionally connected to the wisdom of Earth, a highly developed psychic ability and acute navigational skills in both inner and outer realms; Masculine: centered, grounded, self-responsible, and penetrative	Integration, harmonious balance, peace, radiance, oneness, ease of being, fearlessness	Harmonious balance of masculine and feminine qualities, joy, reunion, full integration—sacred union	Grace, God-reliant, deep-seated ease of being, love, truth, effervescent yet intangibly felt presence	Timelessness, vastness, profound peace, all questions cease to be, all answers found and then tossed aside—the mystery, the gnosis, the unspeakable, the unlearnable, the unknowable

The last three gates are found within the womb and are openings into deeper and more profound intergender healings and corrections. I have discovered that the last three gates are connected to three deep-seated psychic wounds that stretch back as far as the ancient civilizations of Lemuria, Atlantis, and Egypt. It was during these great leaps of consciousness that humankind experienced the deepest injuries between the masculine and feminine polarities. When you read chapter 9 you will discover more in-depth wisdom on this subject and how these same patterns are still playing out to this day in almost every relationship.

THE THREEFOLD
FLAME OF SEXUALITY

As you have read in the beginning pages of this book, we are following the path of the threefold flame because we now know the vital importance of working with three elements in the creation of alchemy. However, within sexuality—the one aspect of the threefold flame that we are covering in this section of the book—we discover the law of three all over again. Within every man and woman there is a sexual trinity of archetypal energies based on the qualities of power, wisdom, and love, which govern and direct sexual expression.

In general most men and women enter blindly into their sexual expression, not knowing that they can change gears and shift qualities of sexual arousal and potentiality. With awareness we can consciously harness and express the core qualities of the archetypal energies found within all human beings. This, in turn, opens us to deeper realms and dimensions of our feminine and masculine essence. Over the course of time human beings have often lost contact with the multitude of realms and dimensions that their soul operates through. However not for one moment did those realms and dimensions ever lose contact with them. It is time for us to remember how to worship the body of the beloved with the full understanding that it is the sacred container of the soul.

Feminine Sexual Archetypes

Assuming that you have integrated Lilith and Eve at the fourth gate, this integrated energy will further evolve into a variety of feminine energy that I am calling the sorceress. This is the archetype that harnesses the reins of your mystical power. Within this trinity we also find the queen, embodying wisdom, and the lover, embodying the flame of love.

By returning to the Star of David formation, we can understand the threefold principle more deeply—the raising of power, the pulling down of wisdom, and the merging in the middle into love. As above, so below.

Within these three feminine sexual archetypes, our goal becomes a balancing of the sacred geometry of the Star of David.

Sorceress: The Flame of Power

Like most things feminine and powerful, the sorceress has been given a bad reputation for being a dark goddess out to seduce and control. Perhaps in some ancient archive of Earth's history that was once the story, but at this time within every conscious woman the sorceress is longing to come forward and bring forth her mystical gifts of magic and transformation. She comes alive with the wild and untameable energy of shakti, the life force, which rhythmically rotates and activates the passions, desires, and physical longing found within a woman. Flowing with shakti, the sorceress is free, unbridled, and at one with all the elements. She is exquisitely aware of the multitude of dimensional realms that she soars through when making love. She can open galaxies and birth new stars with the power of her dreams and intentions. She is found within the first three gates of the yoni: the labia, G-spot, and clitoris, which contain a wild mix of earth, water, and fire. She becomes

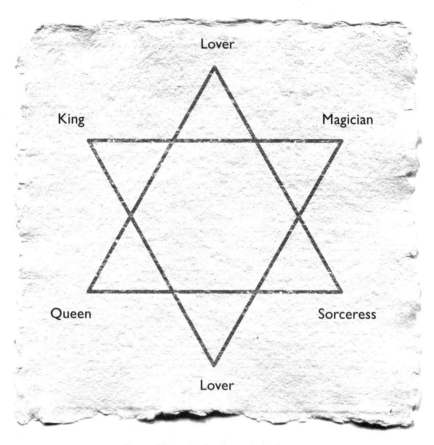

Star of David, the Sexual Archetypes

the spearhead of the lower triangle of the seven gates. When fully cleared, engaged, and consciously taken as a mistress of sacred teachings, the sorceress becomes the voice of the womb of the world, indeed, the spokeswoman for the goddess Gaia.

Her ultimate desire is to meet with the magician, her corresponding archetype found within the masculine.

Queen: The Flame of Wisdom

The queen with her queendom is found inside and through the last three gates of the cosmic womb. She is the spearhead of the upper triangle of the seven gates. The queen is the voice of the heavens, the sovereign of the galactic center. She comes alive with our expansion of consciousness and our resulting ability to see beyond third dimensional reality. Her vision extends through her feminine counterpart as well as her beloved. To open to the archetype of the queen we must delve deep into the fabric of our soul and bring forth the more wild gnostic experiences. Wild gnosis can approximately be described as a direct, transforming experience left untamed and unconditioned by cultural and socioreligious beliefs—the state prior to thought and interpretation of experience, unconfined by concepts and images. Wild gnosis arises in a quiet mind and births from a dimension not touched by chronological time. We find it when we are fully in the present. Not in past or future but here and now. These are the words of the queen as she is the holder of the mystery of Kairos, the sacred present moment.

Her ultimate desire is to meet with the king, the royal archetype of the masculine.

The Lover: The Flame of Love

The lover is found within the fully integrated fourth gate once it is liberated from the push and pull of the light and dark rivers. Once these rivers integrate only one river remains—the river of eternal love. This energy is one of desirous longing and exquisite yearning. The lover archetype is the gateway into extradimensional love. Human beings exist in more than one dimension; we have ten light bodies that connect with the Tree of Life, and these ten light bodies exist in other dimensional spaces. The fourth gate at the entrance to the womb is also known as the anchor point where all dimensions meet and ground in the body.

The fourth gate, once freed from duality and integrated in its polarities, becomes the living heart of the Star of David. This alchemy activates when making love. The fourth gate is also where the masculine leaves his body behind as his fourth gate, the lips of the lingam, kiss the cervix. With the full permission and surrender of the masculine, from this point onward the feminine draws his essence along the length of her fourth gate into and toward the cosmic gates embedded within her womb. This is achieved by a rhythmic pulse that automatically happens with conscious breathing and a clear visualization of the intended act.

The ultimate desire of the feminine lover archetype is to meet with her masculine lover.

Masculine Sexual Archetypes

Once the dark and light rivers of Pan and Christ energy have been integrated in a man at the fourth gate, this combined power will further evolve into a masculine archetype that I am calling the magician. This is the archetype that harnesses the reins of a man's mystical power. Within the threefold trinity of the flames we also find the king, embodying wisdom, and the lover who embodies the flame of love.

If we come back again to the Star of David formation we can see the masculine trinity: the raising of power, the pulling down of wisdom, and the merging in the middle into love. As above, so below.

Magician: The Flame of Power

Unlike his feminine counterpart, the magician has always enjoyed a prestigious place within human history. In England the legendary Merlin, a well-known magician from the times of King Arthur, was famed for his ability to bring forth the mystical gifts of magic and transformation. However, this archetype has become distorted through the patriarchal belief that the magician can only work alone and that a woman may somehow weaken his focus and power. This misperception must be corrected when it exists in the modern-day man, because the magician archetype only comes alive when joined with the wild and untameable energy of the shakti life force from his woman. As she rhythmically rotates and activates her energy, passion, and physical longing for him, he remains still like a pillar, drawing her shakti up into a vertical stream of light. He becomes a pillar, like Shiva—still, eternal, and consistent. In co-creation with the sorceress who opens to the divine flow of shakti, the magician formulates and guides its essence into the alchemical chamber.

The magician is found within the first three gates of the lingam: the perineum, prostate, and length of the lingam, which create a wild mix of earth, water, and fire. He literally becomes the spearhead of the lower triangle of his seven gates. When fully healed and consciously embodied as a master of these sacred teachings, the magician will enable a man to project and penetrate his energy not only in the sexual act but also throughout the inner realms.

His ultimate desire is to meet with the sorceress, the magical archetype found within the feminine.

King: The Flame of Wisdom

The king and his kingdom are found within the hara, located three fingers down from the navel point. This center is also known as the throne of the masculine. The archetype of the king spearheads a man's arrival into the upper triangle of the seven gates found within his woman. The king leads the way along the royal road of the cervix, into the fifth gate of sacred union with the feminine and into the cathedral of light that awaits him in the womb space. To harness the quality of the king one will have to delve deep, and deeper still. The king appears only when you reach and surpass the limits that currently define your life and belief system.

When you meet the king "boy psychology" falls into the unconscious as "man psychology" comes alive.

One of the king's primary functions is to create the transition from boy to man via the means of ordering. The energy of this archetype organizes, orders, and creatively harmonizes all the parts of a man's being. The emergence of the king is profoundly healing and maturing. His energy is creative, generative, and life enhancing. The king becomes the central archetype in the masculine personality around which the rest of the psyche is organized.

Another very important function of the king is to provide fertility and blessing. The king is a conduit for the Divine to pour into man. This is the reason why only the king may ever enter into the womb first. The womb is the infinite well of precreation, and together with the queen, the king sets out to do what he does best—create form, structure, and order from chaos.

His ultimate desire is to meet with the queen, the royal archetype of the feminine.

The Lover: The Flame of Love

The lover is found within the man's fully integrated fourth gate, the lips of the lingam, once he is liberated from the push and pull of the light and dark rivers. In the healed and unified lover, only one river remains: the river of eternal love. This energy is one of a desirous longing to penetrate and enrapture his beloved muse and feminine counterpart. The lover is the gateway into an extradimensional love. For a man as well as a woman it is here at the fourth gate where the anchor point exists to connect and ground all ten dimensions of reality into the body when it is energetically prepared to integrate many dimensions.

Once freed from wounding and duality a man's fourth gate becomes the living heart of the activated Star of David when making love. The fourth gate is where the masculine will leave his body behind as he guides the lips of his lingam to kiss the cervix. From this point onward the feminine will draw his essence along the length of her fourth gate into and toward the cosmic gates embedded within her womb. This is achieved by conscious breathing, a rhythmic pulse that can be felt against the lingam, and by holding a clear visualization of the intended movement of energy. None of this can happen without the full permission and surrender of the masculine. This in itself is a huge initiation as you will be invited to feel and embody the fullness of your surrender. You will be unable to let go and be taken through the sacred doorway if you have any fears or doubts regarding your beloved muse or the feminine principle. Here is where the masculine lover releases himself and becomes the outpouring essence of love, freed from its human bonds. It is here that the lover dies into the arms of his love.

The ultimate desire of the masculine lover is to meet with his eternal muse, the feminine lover.

STAR OF DAVID MERKABA

The word *merkaba* is a Hebrew word (derived from the consonantal root that means "to ride") that describes the throne chariot of God. Throughout the Hebrew, Gnostic, and Christian Bibles we come across this term precisely forty-four times in each edition.

History has talked about the merkaba mostly as the vehicle that allows a person to ascend or descend into the higher or lower worlds, but actually it is much more than only a vehicle of ascension. Its sacred geometry is the primal pattern that created all things and all universes, both visible and invisible. As such, it is one of the blueprints for creation.

In ancient Egypt this primal pattern was called the *mer-ka-ba*. It was actually three words, not one. *Mer* meant a kind of light that rotated within itself. *Ka* meant spirit, in this case referring to the human spirit. And *ba* meant the human body, though it also could mean the concept of reality that spirit holds. And so the entire word in ancient Egypt referred to a rotating light that would take the spirit and the body from one world into another.

In the modern world there are teachers worldwide who are helping people remember the mer-ka-ba. Many of these are the ancients returned at this time to teach a process in consciousness that will eventually transfer us from the third dimensional world into the next higher one through what is being called ascension.

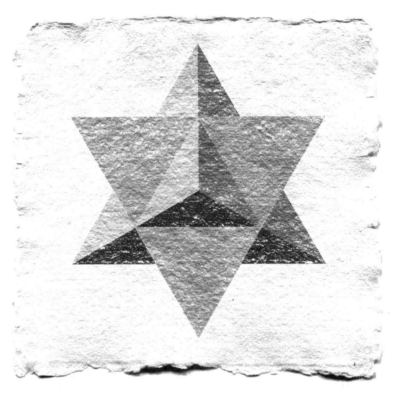

Star of David, Merkaba

Ascension involves a process where the human body is transformed into light and transferred through an incredible birth into a new world. It is achieved through a meditation that requires the mind, heart, body, and spirit to completely integrate in one pattern of light and transcend the human limitations of this reality.

In the context of sacred sexuality, the vehicle of the Star of David Merkaba will be used to:

* merge the upper and lower energies of our seven gates
* heal every aspect of sexuality in all seven gates
* open, clear, and heal all the connecting light channels
  (*nadis* and chakras), which will be used in the first step
  of sacred union

◈ Creating the Star of David Merkaba

■ Individual Practice

Bring yourself into a comfortable seated position with a straight spine, elongated neck, and relaxed, open shoulders, neck, and jaw. Gently press your thumb pads against your first and second fingers creating what is known as the golden triangle in the Kabbalah.

Drop your consciousness into your hips, pelvis, and reproductive system. Breathe deeply into that area, releasing all tensions and nervous energy. Allow the muscular system to relax, the skeletal system to tenderly open, and feel the abundance of the life force begin to freely gather once the container relaxes.

Take your time—spend a good three minutes simply breathing long and deep through your nose, with your eyes closed.

Surrender your awareness deeper still into the first three gates, feeling the three elements of earth, water, and fire. Spend time at each gate, using the breath to relax and open. Imagine that you are guiding life force into every gate with your exhale. The more you breathe, the more vital you become. Begin to sense the arousal of the magician for men and the sorceress for women. Feel them coming alive inside you. Enjoy their wild nature, their limitless and unbridled joy, as they travel through all of life creating magical worlds and experiences. Spend a couple of minutes freely experiencing the energies of the magician and the sorceress.

With great ease, gently begin to gather all the energies of the first three gates into an upward-facing pyramid (see the shape as three dimensional) as this shape becomes the mer, the first part of the sacred geometry.

Bring the qualities of the magician or sorceress to the apex of this pyramid so they spearhead the upward movement.

Gently move your awareness into the upper three gates. Men will now be focusing on the hara—three fingers below the naval point. Women will now be diving with their sensory awareness into the fifth, sixth, and seventh gates inside the womb.

Men, now use your consciousness to ignite the age-old potent powers of the hara, the source point in shamanism. Spend a couple of minutes breathing here as you rouse the energies. Then, begin to feel the qualities of the king in this area of your body.

Women, continue using the breath to expand and open and connect with the qualities of the queen within these extradimensional gates in the womb. As you breathe and waken these archetypal energies, spend time becoming familiar with the qualities of the king or queen. Feel them come alive inside you.

Once a woman has felt the life force of the queen activate, she must also use the three inner womb gates to open her connection to the galactic center—the rotating black hole found in the center of our Milky Way.

Once a man has connected with the king, he must activate his cosmic connection by linking with the central sun, an energetic sun located behind our physical sun.

Remember, as above, so below. Energy follows thought, so use your awareness and breath to do this. Stay seated in your upper gates as you begin to expand outward toward the greater galactic masculine/feminine principles that surround us.

Now just as you did with the first pyramid, merge all the energies of the cosmic womb or hara together into a downward-facing pyramid with the queen or king leading the way and spearheading the descending pyramid. This creates the ba of the sacred geometry.

By using your breath, intention, and visualization, draw the two pyramids together toward the fourth gate. See and feel the creation of the third element—a diamond—being birthed as they first merge into another. This is the creation of ka at the fourth gate.

It is important to feel the anchoring and grounding point of the fourth gate, the place where the two pyramids penetrate one another. This sensation pulls all these energies into your body/consciousness for you to heal, clear, and open. At first this sensation may be painful and emotional to experience. This is perfectly natural and part of the healing experience. You have full permission to respond any way you feel. Please do not hold back your genuine response to this work.

These energies most likely have had their connections and matrixes dulled due to nonuse, so when we do this practice for the first couple of times there could be some surprising results! You are bringing together the correct energetic template for the whole man and the whole woman with a sexual center that is embraced, valued, and rendered sacred.

This truly is a time of celebration!

Continue for eleven minutes. It takes eleven minutes for a human being to be able to consciously stimulate the emotional body and thereby to access any subtle emotional residue in the seven gates.

■ Working Together

When you are exploring together with your beloved on this path, creating the Star of David Merkaba within yourselves before you make love is a very powerful and sacred practice. Each of you creates the merkaba inside before you come together. Before making love take some time to close your eyes, breathe, and consciously create the sacred geometry, again making sure that the merging happens at the fourth gate in both genders. When this becomes second nature you can create the merkaba within seconds. When you both feel ready enter into the experience of making love while gently holding the sacred geometry inside. Be aware of all that is taking place on a much wider scale. Allow yourself to truly drop into the experience, opening your extradimensional sensory awareness. Do not be afraid to feel the deep emotions as they release and also the increasing waves of love that will begin to be entered into. This is all part of the healing and opening journey. Before you begin take some time to connect in prayer in a sincere and pure way as we need to consciously connect with the Divine if we are to emotionally develop and progress from the lover dimensions of sexuality into a more refined expression.

When the time is right, record your discoveries and adventures.

Be prepared! When you begin to experience making love with conscious access to other dimensions and realms, you may become overwhelmed and surprised by just how different all this feels. So my advice to you is to go slowly, pause when you need to, breathe even more deeply, and remember your innate ability to use sound to release and heal. As you clear old energetic blocks give yourself permission to use the other aspect of your expression—your throat. Both fourth gates are powerfully connected to our throats and communication. In fact the size and shape of a woman's cervix will be a mirror image of her cervical vertebrae; even the name gives away the connection!

Remember to use the power of sound! It is the original vibration of creation.

I am sharing this practice with you because it is the most powerful form of subtle light healing that I have come across. This sacred geometry cleanly activates and opens the minute light channels inside the seven gates and the light centers of the ovaries/testes and yoni/lingam.

So, dear dedicated friends, this is our first step: to consciously and emotionally heal our sexuality with all the methods available to us. The creation of the merkaba is a healing of light (masculine), while the seven gates is a healing of love (feminine). Make sure that both partners use both these practices, as these are our inner and outer ways of working with the masculine and feminine principles to effect transformation. We are not using the merkaba at this stage to "travel," only to move and activate energies.

THE HEALING JOURNEY

The sexual healing journey is undertaken first with your own consciousness, and this means that for the most part it is an inner journey with yourself. By all means be loving and intimate with your partner, but I do strongly advise no sex while you are moving through the paths within. A good idea would be to spend one lunar cycle holding back from sex and delving deep into your own relationship with your sexuality and gender. It will be in the next chapter when we do the work together.

If you are working with the template of a lunar cycle (thirty days), you would work with one gate for four days before moving on to the next one. The first and last days would act as introductory and integration days. Make sure that you practice the merkaba visualization at least once while you are working with the gates so that every gate receives the activation that the merkaba will naturally bring.

If you are already in a partnership it would be valuable to share and openly reveal your discoveries. No doubt some huge healings would take place for both of you. However, this must be done by mutual inspiration and agreement. For the most part this is deep and private work, and you will need to give yourself permission to be able to safely dive deep into the old patterns and memories of any and all forms of sexual abuse and projection that you may have experienced as a child.

Sacred Initiation

Take your time as you consciously move through the gates using the Star of David Merkaba exercise above. I would suggest, as there are seven gates, to take seven weeks, focusing on one gate per week. Taking the time to meditate, pray, dance, write, and give every expression imaginable to the voices within them. Your task is to clear your sexuality of all injuries and painful memories regarding sex, shame, guilt, and abuse.

Your dedication is to finally heal and correct any deep-seated resistances and resentments you may have toward the opposite gender—every single one of them. Leave no stone unturned in your search for the Divine and your original innocence. This includes any sexual initiations that you may have received from gurus or Tantra teachers. *Any* sexual act that did not have the fullness of sincere and pure love and connection would have scarred us emotionally. These pastures as well as any surgery or medical examinations or experiences during childbirth, both as a child and a mother, have to be ventured into. Men and woman carry these deep wounds around sexuality, and it is so necessary that we clear them before entering sacred union, otherwise they come up and may unconsciously sabotage the process.

Get yourself a special diary to record your work, especially the voices of the seven gates. Keep this work hidden away unless you consciously choose to share parts of it—you need to feel completely safe within your inner sanctum.

Both partners *must* do this work.

Here is one of my own prayers that could be used for this work. I used it to fully uncover my sexual wounds that I had disconnected from.

> *Dear Mother Father God,*
> *I pray to you with the sincere pure longing within my soul*
>   *to reach and connect with you, my Creator. I humbly*
>   *pray to receive your divine love into my soul as I*
>   *venture into dark pastures of my past as I reclaim my*
>   *consciousness concerning these events.*
> *Please God, please fill me with your divine truth so I may*
>   *fully come to realize and feel what happened. I cannot*
>   *do this without you, [Mother/Father—your choice].*
> *Help me to connect with my true feelings around this*
>   *incident so I may wash clean the error from within*

*my soul, so I may authentically be able to one day
truly connect with my soul half in the masculine form
without carrying this injury.*

*Dear Mother/Father, it is my sincere prayer to become
whole and innocent again, so I may shine forth your
love and truth everywhere within my life.*

*I truly love you with my whole heart and rejoice for the day
when I know that I am with you constantly.*

Amen.

I move forward with trust and consciousness.

3

SACRED SEXUALITY

Tell me friends—is there one among you who would not
awake from the slumber of life if love touched your soul
with its fingertips?
Who among you would not sail the distant seas, cross the
deserts and climb the top most peak to meet the woman
whom his soul has chosen?
What youth's heart would not follow to the ends of the
world the maiden with the aromatic breath, sweet voice
and magic soft hands that had enraptured his soul?
What being would not burn his heart as incense, before
God who listens to supplications and grants his prayer?

KAHLIL GIBRAN,
"AT THE DOOR OF THE TEMPLE"

The essence of this chapter can be sensed in the above quotation from
Kahlil Gibran. In many ways we are now standing at the entrance to
the temple. Here is where we fully engage the first step toward sacred
union. Even though this chapter is devoted to sexuality, this is *not*
the sacred union process; until we reach the end of this book we are

still walking the path of full preparation to enter such an initiation.

This first step, which in itself contains many smaller steps, is the conscious entrance into the first aspect of the threefold flame—*power*. This power is the fullness of your sexuality. Now that you have moved through the seven gates individually, you and your beloved are ready to merge your sexual energies to creatively forge a vessel, a container that will act as a powerful anchor for both of you. This conduit will ground the energies as you proceed through sexual union toward the divine union of heart and soul.

In this first step the sexual act becomes a process of igniting the energetic pathways of the seven gates, leading toward the grand opening of the womb—the cosmic keeper of the grail. Because it is a gateway to profound realms and dimensions, the womb births new codes of evolution and progressive patterns of development into the human collective consciousness. In my opinion the womb births states of consciousness that actually shift the collective field. Therefore it is through women that the more elevated and conscious developments of our species shall be birthed. A man will be able to foresee the intelligence needed for our progression, but until he is in sacred union with a woman, his rate of progression will never know the speed and grace that is possible when they are together. The feminine principle is designed to ground, embody, and bring to Earth. When a woman consciously attends to this process, the results are awe inspiring.

When two people come together consciously, after the process of healing and igniting the seven gates as well as authentically transforming all gender wounds, then for the first time on Earth, they can truly meet in sexual union *exactly* as we once did in the metaphorical Garden of Eden. The threefold flame (power, love, wisdom) is the map of how to return to the living Garden of Eden, which has not gone anywhere, despite the eons we have been lost in separation since the Fall. Despite the tremendous ramifications of not embracing the feminine principle for so long, the garden still patiently awaits us. Deep inside we all feel an intensely lonely longing to apply the healing balm of love to our shared wounds and loss and return home.

If we fell together from the Garden of Eden, then surely it is together that we shall return. As we ate from the apple of wisdom (Sophia) we were granted the experience to know what the gods and goddesses know—that the nature of existence is both light and dark. In my opinion this is the same path that Sophia took, hence the apple being a symbol for wisdom. Sophia, the incarnate God the Mother, descended to Earth to save each and every one of her children, all human souls, from any further suffering and ignorance. However, during her descent she became disconnected and blinded to her true magnificence and lost her way back home.

Like us, she temporarily forgot who she was.

In the gnostic story of Sophia we are told that God the Father sent forth the Logos, the beloved aspect of himself, to find Sophia and to reunite with her in sacred union so that they could both return home, and the heavens could be filled with the presence of the Holy Sophia once again.

In my understanding of "as above, so below" this story clearly shows us the way back home—be it Eden, paradise, or nirvana. The way is sacred union.

THE GUARDIANS OF SACRED UNION

There are two guardians that stand at the entrance of sacred union. One guardian contains the gateway into feminine initiation while the other leads toward masculine liberation. You will have to move through these guardians three times during the entire process. These guardians not only protect the *power* of sexual union but also guard the other two aspects of the threefold flame, *wisdom and love*. Walking this path and confronting the guardians leads to the full expression of emotional bonding and eventually the complete merging of souls.

Every time we experience them, the penetrative process is deeper and stronger, until we have become truly liberated of our greatest fear. They stand guard for two reasons. The first reason is to determine who shall or shall not enter the process. Only the worthy and only the brave shall pass through these guardians, as the fearful presence of what has to be transformed is usually enough to send many running in the opposite direction.

Second, the guardians fiercely protect those who have entered the process, keeping at bay any contrary energies, both internal and external, that may attempt to disrupt the process.

The Fear of Abandonment: The Feminine Guardian

Inside the feminine principle there is a deep and eternal wound—the fear of abandonment by the masculine. Both men and women can access this fear, yet the woman feels the enormity of its depth. For the feminine this fear is not simply the fear of being mildly abandoned or left by her lover. No, the full velocity of this fear is of abandonment throughout all time and space—a wild, cold, and lonely free falling through the cosmos with no hope of ever stopping.

The idea and feeling of entering into the depths of sacred union will release this fear in both of you as you begin the journey. But it will be the woman who takes on the transformation of this initiation as she nears the threshold of bonding so deeply with another. As you move through the passageway of sexual union this fear will have a particular flavor and it will be slightly different each time it arises in the heart and soul.

The fear stems from a deep recessive memory in the feminine psyche that both men and women can access. This place remembers and holds the emotional wounds of the severe disconnection from the masculine. We find this particular story woven into the fabric of the ancient civilization of Lemuria as well as in the portrayal of creation found in *The Right Use of Will* series by Ceanne DeRohan.

We shall be consciously accessing these emotional memories in part 2.

The Fear of Being Consumed: The Masculine Guardian

Deep inside the masculine principle there is a deep and disintegrating fear of being consumed by the feminine to the point of losing identity for good. Again both men and women can access this fear, but it will be the man who will be able to feel the cold terror of its grip. For the masculine this is not a sense of being mildly overwhelmed by the presence of the feminine—it is the eternal dread of being lost, swallowed, consumed to the point of no known return. It is a fear of the absolute annihilation of his identity.

The idea and feeling of entering into the depths of sacred union will release this fear in both of you as you begin the journey. But it will be the man who takes on the transformation of this initiation as he nears the threshold of bonding so deeply with another. As you move through the passageway of sexual union, this fear too will have a particular flavor, and it will be different each time as it arises in the heart and soul.

This fear is rooted in a deep recessive memory in the masculine psyche, which both men and women can access. This ancient place remembers and holds the emotional wounds of a severe disconnection from the feminine. For so long the masculine has endured an existence with the marginalized presence of the feminine. Now that the Goddess is returning, so returns and arises the fear of her overwhelming presence. We find this particular story woven into the fabric of the ancient civilization of Egypt as well as in the portrayal of creation in *The Right Use of Will* series mentioned above.

As you approach sacred sexuality, which is part of the preparation for sexual union, it becomes only a matter of time before these fears will arise. The closer you come together, the more intensely the memories shall surface. It is a good thing to let it happen in full consciousness; in fact, I am positively encouraging you to enter the process.

I invite you both to authentically feel into these fears when you are alone or together through the use of guided meditation or journeywork. For a woman the roots of the abandonment can be found in her lower body, usually the first root chakra, while for a man the fear of being consumed is located in his third eye and upper body. To begin the transformation process you will be looking to share intimately with one another the nature of these fears in a vulnerable and authentic way. Openly reveal any emotions and thoughtforms associated with the fears. This intimate exchange needs to take place in a sacred setting where both people feel safe and held so that the deep secrets of the psyche can arise innocently with no judgment and no need or desire to be fixed. This is just a simple confession of what is being discovered inside and a sacred offering toward becoming vulnerable and transparent with one another.

I must repeat again—you are not trying to fix or heal these fears in one another. No attempt to make them go away is required! The purpose of this work is to:

* connect to the fears
* use your feminine principle to feel them in your body
* use your masculine principle to witness them in your consciousness
* confess with vulnerability, tenderness, and authenticity to your beloved, revealing fully the nature of the fear and how it plays out in your day-to-day life
* share the deep, nostalgic threads of your soul memories

The great work is performed when you are consciously able to connect to these fears and bring them into the lovemaking process.

Therefore a woman will be connected to the fear of abandonment while receiving the fullness of her man in a raw, potent, present, and deeply committed way. While the man (during a different intimate time) will connect to the fear of being consumed while surrendering with penetration into the great abyss with the full presence of his woman in a raw, potent, and deeply committed way. This experience creates an exquisite paradox that over time will transform the fear completely.

One more thing we have to realize here is that the area of sacred sexuality is usually where the woman experiences the deepest healings and releases. In general it is the feminine that experiences the profundity of sacred sexuality, while it's the masculine that receives the greatest breakthroughs with the soul consciousness work (in the later chapters). Women in general have withheld the fullness of their sexuality, while men in general have withheld their inner world. These are intergender injuries of ancient Egypt that play out to this day. We shall be covering these injuries in love as we dive deeper into the book.

It is important that the woman feels able to access the fear and to authentically express from deep within the experience. A man must be able to stay present during his exposure to the emotions, cries, words of anguish, and possible contortions of pain within her body or in her facial gestures. A man must compassionately realize the enormity of this pain, which is as old as time itself. As I said—this is the great work.

The man is invited to enter into the great abyss as he begins to make love, bringing with him the fear that he is going to become lost by the overwhelming presence of his woman, that he may well be consumed by his love for her. He is being invited to feel into his complete loss of identity, into the fear that he will become nullified throughout all time and space, lost in the nothingness, in the void herself. To reconcile the paradox here a man must master the art of surrender. As he surrenders completely to the void he will begin to enter the transformation process. It is important that the man feels able to access his fear and to authentically express from deep within the experience. A woman must be able to stay present, exposed to his emotions, his cries, his words of anguish, and the possible contortions of pain within his body or on his face. The woman too must realize with compassion the enormity of this pain that is as old as time itself.

Another way to open these stories more fully is by listening to them on my *Wounds of Love* album, although the transcript is presented here in chapter 9. In my album I provide you with guided journeys, which are designed to lead you toward the innermost parts of your being where the psychic memories of the personal and collective intergender wounds reside. To know love, to truly touch its depths, we must let go of all our guards and drop with totality into our own vulnerability.

Please note that it is important to keep reading until the end of this chapter before you make love with penetration for the first time. You must read through and prepare for the sacred initiation at the end of this chapter before you complete the exercises laid out below. The first time is hugely important with regard to time and space, as its sets in motion the law of cause and effect. If you are wise you will give your consummation the fullness of your attention and foresight. If you have already made love and consummated your relationship (and there are many who have!), you can consciously choose again by applying this wisdom to initiate a second consummation date. You cannot erase the creation of your first coming together, but you can bring the fullness of your intention to create a new chapter in your relationship.

SACRAMENTS OF SACRED UNION

The word *sacrament* means "sacred oath" and is often viewed as an outward and visible ceremony that is a reflection of the inward and spiritual divine grace that is being consciously embodied. It is with this kind of reverence that we begin the next part of our journey. As we enter the full sacred union process we shall be bringing forth the seven sacraments, which are similar to the oaths taken in the Christian faith as well as other religions. The performing of ritual and ceremony is an aspect of life that has nearly been wiped out in the modern Western world. In order to balance humankind with Earth once again rituals and conscious ceremonies must be engaged in. Recently there has been profound change and transformation in regard to the understanding of this. I offer the seven sacraments as a further step in the healing that ritual brings to Earth and her people. These sacraments are based on sacred union. They minister to the body, heart, and soul and lead them to their original creation blueprint, which includes the reunion of twin souls, the harmonization of opposites, and atonement with God.

As we progress through the preparation stages I feel it is important that we embrace the elements of ritual and ceremony so that we can begin to work with the Divine Feminine in a fresh way, welcoming her back into our lives as the representative of sacred work.

Let us begin with the sacrament of the body. This is the first step in sacred sexuality and is symbolized by the flame of power. The moment you and your beloved begin to enter through the seven gates together by the penetrative process of sexual intercourse you are committing both of your bodies exclusively to each other and to the process. It is my very deep knowing that no other can enter this space of deep communion with you. This means there must be no other man or woman on the sidelines, no sexual projection onto another, no third party coming in via any other means from pornography to flirtatious exchanges online. The backdoor of your sexual exchanges needs to be firmly closed for this sacrament to work alchemically. We will be unable to give our fullness to one another if we are always ready to leave at the slightest test or challenge.

When our spiritual centers open to their full extent we will easily be able to see the leaks in ourselves and in our partners, but up until then our own integrity and sense of honor must attend to the matter. Sever all connections with other people of the opposite sex who wish to engage with you sexually or emotionally in a manipulative way. We must see to it that our primary connection is with our partner and not our mother or father. The man *has* to disconnect from his mother and place his beloved in the primary feminine role, while the woman has to do the same thing regarding her father. These are giant steps that need to be taken for this to authentically move to the next level. Energetically this sacred act can only take place once we close the backdoor and cast instead a sacred circle.

If you are having a problem with this and are feeling a sense of resistance, pause and give this resistance your greatest attention. We must be fully committed every step of the way and should only proceed when we experience the warm emanation of our true happiness and hunger to proceed. Whenever we experience a knot of tension we must pause and examine. This is the body's way of telling us attention is needed.

Never allow your partner to persuade you to move forward if you are not ready. It takes a mature conscious examination to reach the purity of truth woven into your internal sensations and messages. Finally, be honest at least with yourself. Use a journal to write down your discoveries and openly confess to yourself. Better still, tenderly share with your partner your discoveries with a sensitivity and delicateness that encourages him or her to stay open and receptive. The reason I use the word *confess* is that its true meaning is to disclose something that is damaging or inconvenient to oneself or another. When a full confession has been genuinely given and received both parties will experience a deep relaxation and the ability to go to the next level in intimacy and connection.

When you are ready to truly proceed know that the first time you make penetrative love you are offering all of your body. Be sure to realize this in the act of making love, and give yourself fully. Connect with every heartbeat, every breath, every wave of emotion felt through the body, every ripple of movement, every touch of your hands and tongue. Every kiss, every glimpse of one another through effulgent eyes, every caress, every gasp for air, every bead of sweat. Build and build the furnace of your passion, leave no stone unturned as you search for more of your beloved everywhere.

Use your body to bring into manifestation the fullness of your love for your partner. Let every stroke whisper with your longing, every expansion of your iris bring through more light, let every brush of your lips administer the healing nectar of reunion. Imagine—for it may well be true—that you have been separated for eons, throughout all time and space, and that this moment has been given to you so that you may discover one another again in the flesh.

Let every moment count as you consciously release any polite constraints you may have bound yourself with. Dissolve your prison walls, knowing that there is nowhere you cannot go and nothing you cannot express. Bring your fears and resistances to the furnace of your fiery passion, burn everything in sight that attempts to self-sabotage and manage this love in nice little doses. Let this love run free and wild across the terrain of your lives, pulling up and tearing apart the hopeless constraints of mind and its attempts to keep this love simmering rather than enticing this rapture to explode throughout all existence.

This is what I mean when I say give your body.

THE LOVER'S PATH

When you have moved through the seven gates by yourself and reconnected to the energies of all seven voices (see previous chapter), the next step is to take the journey with your beloved. The lone path allows you to personally transform the wounds that you may discover along the royal road leading from the yoni to the womb in a woman and from the perineum to the tip of the lingam in a man. You have to become so intimate and familiar with not only your own masculine and feminine principles but also those of your partner. There is an alchemy that takes places when you *fully* know and experience that you are both man and woman in one body. Only then does that wholeness ignite the full path.

> A male is not truly male unless he becomes a full and complete female. A female is not truly female unless she is first fully and completely male. Those who would enter the bridal chamber must be complete in themselves. There are those who try to find their completion in another and I say to you, they deceive themselves. They may search and even think they find, but are never complete in themselves. Unless you are male and female in yourselves, you remain outside of the Eye of the Mystery.
>
> TESTAMENT OF MIRIAM OF MAGDALA,
> FROM *THE GOSPEL OF MARY MAGDALENE,*
> TRANSLATED BY JEAN-YVES LELOUP

Sacrament of the Body

Now as you make love together with awareness of this royal road, you are asked to slow down and to consciously connect with one another's gates before penetration. It is important for both partners to give the threefold attention of passion, love, and inner vision to the first four gates. As each gate meets and touches this attention can be amplified with a loving, penetrating gaze that sees through the flesh into the light codes and geometries within as well as by applying the conscious touch of your fingers, lips, and tongue, enticing your partner to open and trust deeply. Breathing out slowly and deeply with your mouth while carrying a soulful intention to connect with the deep innermost aspects of each gate is a powerful way to connect. Whispering prayers, mantras, and resonant sounds will also help to unlock the mysteries. The anointing of oil into the gateways is a beautiful opening gesture, though you must make sure that the oil is diluted so as not to cause a painful sensation.

Before the man even enters the woman's first gate there needs to be a conscious pause. In this moment he approaches the entrance to her yoni, offering his loyalty and full presence, recognizing the sacredness of this act and feeling the sincere welcome emanating from within her. Once both partners have felt the connection it is up to the woman to give the signal that permission to enter has been granted. She may whisper her invitation to enter, use her hands to guide his lingam, or press against him, causing his lingam to open her.

Both the man and the woman will be consciously connecting to the first four gates inside the woman. The woman will be feeling her man move through and enter the energetic fields of her gates while she is opening ever deeper internally. As he enters her she will perceive him as both form and light. It is important for the woman to become so sensitive in the gates that she actually feels his essence as light, unlocking and activating her gates. Inside every gate there will be a gift, a code just for him, which will both open and adorn him. The man will be aware of connecting with the full presence of his lingam and bringing the energetics of his first two gates into the experience as two rooted, anchoring portals.

Let there be a pause as the fourth gate of the man (tip of the lingam) touches the fourth gate of the woman (tip of the cervix). Over time we need for this moment to become highly sensitive and almost etheric. Ideally the man does not rub up against the side of the cervix but just touches the lips of the lingam on the cervix, kissing the delicate opening at the tip of the cervix, known as the stargate. Linger here for a moment, feeling one another's sexual energies and the aroused state of one another's physical organs. Let the fourth gates come to know one another as they consciously meet for the first time. This sacred touch is the key that unlocks the power of the threefold flame. The masculine is invited at this moment to become brilliantly aware of the light that he is bringing to the darkness of the great womb. He is truly bringing forth the light of the sun/son, the solar essence, into the black light of the grail space. The touching of the fourth gates is a glorious moment in which you both can hold space and witness internally the beauty of this divine alchemy. This is a very significant moment, a prelude to the point at which the man will leave behind his physical body and allow his essence to be drawn through the woman's fourth gate toward the magnetic pull of the womb, bringing his light with him.

This inner movement through the fourth gate can happen only with the conscious intent of the woman to fully receive him into the womb space and with the man's conscious surrender to that magnetic receptivity in the womb space. The woman uses her breath and visualization to draw him up through the center of her cervix, connecting to the desirous longing of her heart for him to touch her in the deepest, innermost places. The woman is required in time to reveal and open every part of her sexual nature, leaving nothing hidden for herself. This experience takes time and does not need to be rushed or forced in any way.

The man will be connecting at this time to his surrender and his ability to truly let go of his mind and his structured form. He will merge with his surrender and his desire and enter into the great abyss of the love and desire emanating from his woman and the fullness of the Divine Feminine pulsating through her. At this gate the man takes an energetic leap of faith as he consciously chooses to travel through the cervix toward the womb, leaving his identity behind and entering the innermost temple of creation, the ever beckoning, pulsating sanctuary of life and death. In this moment he surrenders to becoming pure light. It is toward these tremendously powerful archetypal paradigms that he is heading. It is almost as if the feminine is waiting for him at the top of the cervix, he has to travel this part alone to crystallize his intent and rite of passage.

As you both begin to feel the warm, fluid opening of the fifth gate at the neck of the cervix into the vastness of the womb, that is the sign to merge at an even greater depth. The fact that the woman can feel her man's essence at her fifth gate should be all it takes to recognize the nobility of his prayerful intention that his journey toward her is strong and committed. She must allow the deep reaches of his presence to open her heart and soul as she receives him into her innermost chambers.

It is up to the expert guidance of the woman to delicately guide the waves of intense love radiating from her heart down toward her womb. This potent alchemy of devotional love and power (shakti and bhakti in Sanskrit terminology) is also known as the fountain of youth, and it has the power to rebirth your beloved. In the Egyptian Mysteries we are told that the love of a woman goddess has the power to resurrect her beloved from the dead as well as bring about a profound rebirth for her man. (I have experienced this directly myself.)

After the fifth gate opens continue the process of guiding the masculine toward the sixth and seventh gates as he surrenders deeper and deeper into the energies that will be starting to permeate his consciousness. These energies will be a rising of the womb of the world, the pulsation of Gaia herself as well as a downpouring from galactic center, our human birthing portal onto planet Earth. Women, hold these truths inside! The more deeply you connect to your sixth and seventh gates through meditation and lovemaking (especially afterward when you are in the nesting phase) the more profoundly they will reveal the truths of your connection to the triple goddess who manifests as your womb, the planetary womb, and the galactic womb—maiden, mother, and crone. Remember that the sixth gate holds the codes and blueprints as to why you and your beloved have found one another. Inside the sixth gate will be the reason and purpose of your union. You both must locate, access, and open that seed code. With the woman's guidance the man can penetrate the code with his light, and the woman can sense internally the information as a spectrum of feelings and visions.

Once the man reaches the energetic depths of the womb space the energies within will configure to accept and hold the sacred geometry of his masculine essence. She becomes his. That is why it is impossible for another man to enter her womb when a woman is on the sacred union path of initiation. The womb simply will not allow another man to come forward in any way.

This means that every time the man enters his beloved's womb space this geometry is there to greet him after spending deep and rich time in the grail space since he last left. This is why the woman always feels as if he is inside her and that their connection is eternal, as she is indeed carrying his essence.

In this profound lovemaking you can choose to orgasm or not. Some people choose to save their orgasm and channel the energies through the spine toward the sacred glands in the head to replenish and expand their spiritual bodies. However, if you are opting to orgasm then the ideal conclusion would to be to orgasm together.

The other way to replenish your energies after orgasm is for you both to drop into the womb space and beyond. It has been my experience that access to the rich depths that pulse from within the timeless resonance of the womb space is far greater after orgasm, causing both people to pass out or lose consciousness after making love. However, in my recent explorations I am discovering that this deep space doesn't always necessarily rely upon orgasm. So in essence this is something for you to genuinely explore for yourselves.

COCOONING

The transition from movement to stillness is an essential part of the replenishing or restoration process. In the ancient texts this period is known as the resurrection and/or rebirth of the masculine. From deep within the womb space an even stronger magnetic field begins to unfold and slowly rotate around the two beloveds, encapsulating and bringing into unison the ten light bodies of each person. This mirrors precisely the essential nature of our galactic center with its infinite black hole beckoning all life toward its ultimate surrender into the great pull of the void.

This is where the masculine shall meet an even greater aspect of his fear, for here is where he is being called to enter. To lie within his woman's arms and surrender to his mortal beloved is one step; entering into the colossal depths and rivers of her eternal being is a different matter altogether. Of course we have to remember that this will mirror the same process for the masculine principle within the woman. A woman with a strong masculine side may also experience fear as she drops ever deeper into the surrender of her feminine being rather than following the impulse of doing, which is a natural trait for the masculine.

Yet beyond this veil is where you shall both receive the sacred nectar of your union. When you enter this space, at first you may simply lose consciousness. Its richness and frequency is so exquisitely restoring yet so desperately needed that most of us pass out and regain consciousness sometimes hours later, asking, "What on *Earth* just happened?"

How to Enter Cocooning

Once you have reached orgasm coast inwardly on the energy and don't lose sight of it for a moment. Allow the waves of your internal energies to profoundly unfold, to reveal the furthermost reaches of its exquisite expanse. While gently riding the waves of innermost pleasure, come into a lying position where the man is resting in the woman's arms. This position is called cocooning, also known as nesting or encircling.

Invite the man to become exquisitely comfortable, warm, and relaxed. The woman tenderly begins to drift inward toward her sixth gate, the conception point, bringing awareness to where the spark of life shines, feeling within the raw, potent pulse of creation. She then begins to drop even deeper as she passes through the sixth gate toward the seventh, feeling the gateway that leads from her physical womb into the unseen worlds. A part of her remains at the seventh gate while at the same time becoming absolutely aware of her beloved within her arms. With a minimum of effort she begins to encircle or cocoon her man, gathering his energy within her conscious awareness and then gently drawing him into her womb toward the seventh gate.

I have to share with women the absolute truth: Your womb, your innermost feminine essence, knows exactly how to do this; all you really have to do is drop down into the rich source of your feminine essence and surrender. There really is no doing, just a letting go and allowing your inherent feminine nature to come alive and guide you both into the cosmic womb for restoration, resurrection, and rebirth.

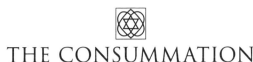

THE CONSUMMATION

The next step is to use the exercises above and sacred initation below to complete the consummation. The word *consummation* means "to complete" or "to finalize." The way we can see this act energetically is by the words and action of "closing the backdoor" and "opening up the sacred circle."

I see the backdoor as a device that many of us have when we are uncommitted and flighty. It is our "get out" clause that keeps the backdoor slightly ajar in case something or someone better comes along. It renders us unable to give our fullness to one another as we always have our eye on the backdoor, always ready and prepared to leave at the slightest test or challenge.

This step is *not* the entrance into sacred union. The consummation of your lovemaking through the seven gates begins to harness the purity found within the spiritual fire of holy sexuality. The deep process of sexual healing and bonding begins with this practice and ultimately culminates in sacred union.

⬡ Sacred Initiation

Remember to choose the right time and place for the first time you make love in trust and consciousness. Below you will find some guidelines.

* Choose the moment wisely—consult the lunar cycle, apply the kabbalistic wisdom, be conscious (avoid full moons, when the moon is waning, and both of your Saturn days and phases).
* Be fully present, no alcohol, drugs, or intoxicants of any kind—not the first time.
* Choose your environment wisely: When you consummate for the first time, you open a portal for all your light bodies to give and receive energy (and your environment becomes part of that

exchange). Intend for your environment to be clear and pure enough to reflect your holy union.

* Enter into a prayerful space, asking God to bless your union.

* Bring yourself fully into the moment: Sit opposite one another and breathe together, maybe exchanging breaths with your mouths (inhaling his breath, and exhaling your own); connect with and amplify your five senses *first* so that you can receive the fullness of one another through these five channels.

* Connect with and stimulate all four gates in one another, knowing that the last three can only be reached through sexual union.

* Build and build your passion for something beyond your relationship, for a dimensional expression way beyond the human experience; keep reaching to experience that original moment when you both came into existence as one soul; don't be afraid of all the feelings that brings up.

* Take your fears of abandonment and being consumed into the bonfire of your desire and longing for one another.

* Finally, sleep together the whole night and try to stay comfortably interwoven. *Do not* leave one another after the sexual act if you have not fallen asleep; you must sleep or at least deeply rest to integrate.

Consummation is the act of stepping over an invisible line. The moment you make love, there will be a huge shift emotionally and energetically. Choose your moment wisely with the mantra of this work:

I move forward with trust and consciousness.

PART TWO

Emotional Intimacy

The Second Trimester

The dust of the earth is the crown you have been looking for your whole life.

BEN BUSHILL, "DUST OF THE EARTH"

4

LONGING

The Sacred Heart

When you are joyous, look deep into your heart and you
shall find it is only that which has given you sorrow
that is giving you joy.
When you are sorrowful look again in your heart, and you
shall see that in truth you are weeping for that which
has been your delight.

KAHLIL GIBRAN, "ON JOY AND SORROW"

As we continue onward and upward with our journey, we take with us all the passionate, creative power of our reclaimed sexuality, tenderly offering its sacredness as we kneel before the altar of our heart.

The second part of this journey has a different terrain and takes on a new tempo. With sexuality the key that unlocked the gates was the pulsating power of shakti, the spark of creativity, the raw essence of life itself. However when we kneel before the heart it is only by the sacred touch of bhakti, a form of devotional love, that such a boundless glory can open. There can be no reserved private space left in our hearts. As

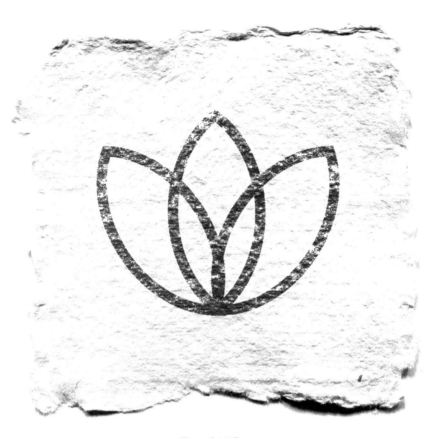

Threefold Flame

we enter this profound shift in our relationships we are being beckoned to fully love being together, treasuring every moment to touch, to see, to breathe, and to sleep together like cuddling field mice. Real purity never gets used to that.

As we approach the real depths of the heart, which we have been longing for all this time, we will discover some initiatory guardians known as the wounds of love. These wounds prevent deeper connection and deeper intimacy. As we turn the pages we will understand more about these wounds, how they can show up and ways to move through them. This shall become our preparatory work toward heartfelt sacred union.

However deeply you feel you have loved in the past, forget it—you are now going to be taken to the next octave. When you enter in to heartfelt union you will go beyond any past limitations. Within the chambers of your heart you shall come to know the many forms of love that emanate from the source. This journey into the heart is exquisite, and for me it was and is the most painful. It is a pain that I would surrender to every day of my precious life—over and over again. Its bittersweet agony is so refreshingly honest as its pain reveals one's own fragility and tenderness. I would often wonder whether *love* was the right word to describe what I felt. The places I would wander into with my beloved were, in some ways, where "we" were not, where absence or vastness was and is. Something greater than the personal opens, burns, and rises through. It cannot be understood or described, but it can be lived.

At the entrance to the heart we find many gathered, all claiming that they have the willingness to enter, all speaking of love and how deeply they are prepared to give their lives to the rapture of becoming this love. But this is not something you become, because it is not just another step along the path; the enormity of this love is the very essence that gave birth to the creation of the path and your own internal longing to walk it. To be a lover, you must lay down all your powers and intellectual learning. Every trophy, every victory, and every wound must be given to the feet of the *one* that breathed life into you. Love asks you to surrender to the mystery of life itself. It takes a special kind of grace to be consciously aware of when we are denying this immense love.

True lovers at the entrance to the heart are the ones who do not stand around talking about it but instead draw a deep breath together, bow their heads in reverence, and walk in naked with their arms outstretched.

For these lovers know that by entering the heart they are entering themselves. They know that every hurt they feel along the way is a blessed obstacle to overcome. All eyes glisten with gratitude as they look toward the fullness of the heart, never turning back to the world for opinion or blame. They know that every wound they stumble onto is from the tender damage of being separated from their beloved while here in the separated human form.

Notice I used the word *beloved* there, leaving the space open for you to interpret who I am referring to. For me the word *beloved* refers to both God and my twin soul. I do not see any separation between them. Finally, I do not see any separation between them and myself. But do you?

Let's explore deeper.

> Love one another, the way I have loved you.
> LAST WORDS OF JESUS CHRIST
> TO HIS DISCIPLES, JOHN 13:34–35

I do not believe that two human souls can successfully walk this path alone without connection to the Divine. I truly believe that sacred union is the path of reunion for twin souls into at-one-ment with God. If you are to travel unprotected into the emotional wounds of the heart you will absolutely need divine assistance. This sacred lineage is one that does not accept justifications, reasoning, excuses, or the sidestepping of issues that arise. It asks us to go beyond merely transcending the pain and to never deny the enormity of the path and lineage that we have chosen. We walk this sacred path not only for ourselves but also for the collective human consciousness. We, the ones who carry the flame of this sacred lineage, shall not accept denial, guilt, or shame as reasons to shut down further exploration. These inner sensations are instead used as our transforming fire in the purest search for truth.

At this time of awakening to the sacred union process the activations and initiations will be occurring at an intense and quickening level. Those of you who are reading this book have chosen to be on planet Earth at this time of awakening, knowing your vibration of high love is birthing a new era of unity consciousness. This means that each individual's consciousness is changing, via the human vessel, throughout all the interconnected ten light bodies.

The core of this energetic vibrational shift is to become whole within. This work of wholeness requires that every once-denied emotional pattern has to be released and brought to the light to be accepted and loved, creating a new paradigm of unconditional love for the *self*, first and foremost.

This new Christ consciousness is the embodiment of the activated twin soul heart of pure balance and empowered abundance within— and therefore without.

There is much confusion at this time regarding the sacred twin soul reunion. This is because the sacred twin soul reunion is of the Christ consciousness and not of the third dimensional vibration of limited mental concepts. As Earth transitions to a higher frequency in her evolutionary expansion, that which seems enigmatic now will become clear.

The true twin soul is your perfect tonal mate, meaning the balanced and opposite intonation of vibration. Your twin soul is matched to you by the laws of creation through harmonics and resonance. One must have a clear energy field, which reflects an inner integration of masculine and feminine, to successfully carry the frequency of full physical sacred reunion with one's twin soul.

This understanding is not from a third dimensional thought perspective but from what I call a gnostic deep knowing. The fullness of your being receives the truth as waves of experience, rather than one-pointed knowledge straight into the mind.

As more and more of you come into this harmonic balance, you will connect with your true twin soul. Many of you have a knowing that this is your unique purpose at this time.

You may wonder how you reach this inner balance of vibration and the frequency of your fullness. I can only answer: Pray with the essence of your heart.

As I have traveled this path and accessed ever deeper aspects of my true nature, I have found myself reverting to good old-fashioned prayer. There is no lasting solace in my old ways of processing emotion. I have reached such depths of sorrow and agonizing aloneness that my heart yearns only for God. Along this pathway I have fallen into the deepest pits of despair, gone to places that no other spiritual path or teacher could have taken me. I have found that only the one who created me has the power and the love to reach me in those dark moments and illumine me with grace. When I have been opened so deeply—through bittersweet, agonizing joy—to see the honest, raw, and naked essence of myself, the only response left is gratitude. In that place, filled with the sweetest waves of humility, there is nothing else, just an eternal and innocent "thank you."

> *Love cannot be described,*
> *It must be tasted.*
>
> RUMI

FIVE FORMS OF LOVE

There are four Greek words for love that are important for us to understand so that we can feel into their different flows and to check that they are running, knowing that they are simply different facets of the one diamond. The Greek words for love are *eros, agape, philia,* and *storge.* However, to complete our path, we also need to add the word *rapture.* Finally, its important to remember that this love is threefold in nature: love for self, other, and God.

Eros

The Greek word for *sexual love* or *passionate love* is "eros," which is the root of English words such as *erotic* and *eroticism*. When eros is used as a proper noun it refers to the Greek god of love, who carries the same name.

Eros is based on strong feelings toward another. It usually occurs in the first stages of a man-woman romantic relationship. This love is based on physical traits and attractions, and it can be based more on what can benefit you rather than the other person. This is "I love you because it feels good and makes *me* happy loving you." See? The key word is the word *me*. When in eros we must become mindful of the change into another form, making sure that the aliveness and evolving nature of love transforms with us. The very essence of love is creative, unexpected, and beautifully unpredictable.

However, bestselling author of spirituality and conscious relationships Marianne Williamson points out that within the initial first flush of romantic eros there is a confluence with the sacred known as the mystery of romance. In her blog she makes the following observation.

> The common wisdom goes like this: that the myth of "some enchanted evening," when all is awash with the thrill of connection and the aliveness of new romance, is actually a delusion . . . a hormonally manufactured lie. That soon enough, reality will set in and lovers will awaken from their mutual projections, discover the psychological work involved in two people trying to reach across the chasm of real life separateness, and come to terms at last with the mundane sorrows of human existence and intimate love. . . . From a spiritual perspective, the original high of a romantic connection is thrilling because it is true. . . . We are having what you might call a mini-enlightenment experience. . . . Our problem is

that most of us rarely have a psychic container strong enough to stand the amount of light that pours into us when we have truly seen, if even for a moment, the deep beauty of another. The problem we have is not that in our romantic fervor we fall into a delusion of oneness; the problem is that we then fall into the delusion of separateness.

Eros, then, can point us to the true reality, which can be sustained only by those willing to heal the blocks of the wounded personality.

Agape

The Greek word that refers to the love of God is *agape*. Agape is the very nature of God, for God is love, absolute divine love. The big key to understanding agape is to realize that it can be known through the very action it prompts. People today are accustomed to thinking of love as a feeling, but that is not necessarily the case with agape. Agape is a form of love that flows because of what it does, what it attends to, and what it transforms, not because of how it feels.

Agape is an exercise of the will, a deliberate choice to align with love. I often use the words *surrender to love* to mean becoming a servant of love; this does not mean sitting in meditation, merely feeling the bliss waves of love. Rather the impulse of agape is found in action—in words and deeds of love. There is a joyful uprising of love, which wants only to give of itself, to pour out into the world its true benevolent force. The feeling is one of joy helplessly overflowing combined with a delight in knowing that you have become bound to love by the relinquishing of your personal will. This living experience of liberation is often called unconditional love. Yet even to put the word *unconditional* in front of love suggests that in our ordinary human experience we know so little of love's essence, value, and inherent power of benevolent transformation and rebirth.

Philia

The third word for love is *philia,* which means to have a special interest in someone or something, frequently with focus on close association, and have affection for, like, or consider someone a friend. Philia refers to a strong liking or a strong friendship, and in our modern vernacular the word has come to mean love. We say we love things that we strongly like: I love ice cream. I love my car. I love the way your hair looks. The word *philia* implies a strong emotional connection, and thus it means the love, or deep friendship, between friends. There is a distinction here—you can agape your enemies, but you cannot philia them.

Storge

The fourth Greek word we need to understand is *storge,* which is the love and affection that naturally occurs between parents and children. This love can exist between siblings, and it exists between husbands and wives in a good marriage. It is a form of brother-sister love, and it is crucial to reach this love before the sacred union process. We need to be able to feel the absolute trust and deep friendship that kind of bond creates for the process to deeply integrate.

Here is where we find the terms *sister bride* and *brother groom.*

Rapture

I wish to include the word *rapture,* which means the heightened state of being lifted up, almost transfigured, as Christ was in raising his light body. With the word *rapture* there is a sense of teleportation and being uplifted into a devoted, ecstatic state.

This rapture is a form of love. I have only experienced this in profound states of God realization, unspeakable beauty, fathomless flows of love, immense gratitude, and overwhelming longing for something that you know you already have. It is so tangible; it can actually give the impression of hurting the body as its enormity of charge passes through the finite chamber of the human form. The transportation is toward the source of love—God, the Source, whatever you wish to call our Creator. When this happens nothing else exists, nothing else matters. We become devoted, enraptured, and transported to a time and space way beyond our ordinary understanding.

These five distinct types of love are discovered *within* the wounds of love once we have worked through them. They also relate to the five fundamental elements of humankind: betrayal conceals eros, separation conceals agape, denial conceals philia, judgment conceals storge, and abandonment conceals rapture. In essence, eros is sexual, agape is spiritual, philia is emotional, storge is physical, and rapture is soulful.

To enter the fullness of sacred union it becomes essential to first understand these aspects of love and to sense your affinity with them within your day-to-day experiences. Second, it is important to clear any emotional or spiritual reasons, or possible contracts or vows, that may have kept you from experiencing each type of love. It is vital that these channels of love are discovered, cleared, and ready to become used in the most joyful of ways.

So let's do a quick check.

1. Do you access sexual vitality and passion for your partner? Can you feel passionate and sensual? Are you able to be moved by powerfully evocative love stories, songs, and poetry?
2. Do you access unconditional love and become moved to contribute toward a group or community? Do you, or could you, welcome the whole world into your heart and home?
3. Do you really love your friends and have passion for spending time with them, deepening your relationship? Are you in love with activities and passions? Do you, or can you, weep when you experience either touching moments or forms of suffering in others?
4. Do you love your family? Do you enjoy being with them? Are

there any unhealed, unloving relationships within the family? Are there any family feuds?

5. Do you love God with your whole heart, and do you have a personal relationship with the Divine? Can you feel the love of God move through you? Can you feel devotion fill your heart in forms of ecstatic worship and honoring of your God?

THE SENSE OF LONGING

In my understanding the sweet essence of sorrowful longing abundantly arises within the feminine heart. I say sorrowful because this particular frequency is a bittersweet one, paradoxically aching with joy to love ever deeper, ever wider. At its essence the yearning of longing wants to extend, to reach out and toward, and yet at the very same time, it desires to deeply receive. If one can stay with this delicious pain of longing it actually fulfills itself, and one reaches the heart of the beloved within. However, many people resist getting fully into a state of longing, afraid of its enormity and out-of-control nature. It is true. Longing is totally wild, untameable, and wonderfully unpredictable. It will take you hostage—and release you like a plaything when the mystical kiss has been received. Only one who has surrendered can live the ecstatic mystery of longing.

When I was in Assisi, Italy, I read the letters of Saint Clair, who founded the feminine order of nuns alongside Saint Francis's order of monks. Saint Clair's letters to Agnes of Prague are aflame with a passion that sits easily alongside Rumi. In their unbridled longing they helped me to find another piece in the puzzle of love's alchemy, because for many years I had sensed that this kind of wild longing was a key element in sacred union, and that this path was not for the fainthearted but for the ones willing to burn with holy desire. Another piece dropped into place and my suspicion was overwhelmingly confirmed the first time I experienced a Gnostic Mass of the

Holy Order of Mary Magdalene. Within moments of entering into the ceremony I was filled with a crystal-clear clarity that proclaimed that longing and gratitude are the two key ingredients that alchemically activate the third element—rapture.

Whenever feminine longing and masculine gratitude enter the heart at the same time and hold those paradoxical opposites in union, the result is the ignition of a rapture, which raises one in divine ecstasy, rendering one speechless.

I had finally found the alchemical sequence to unlock the heart.

> *Draw me after you, Heavenly Spouse,*
> *for we shall run in the fragrance of your perfumes!*
> *I shall run and not grow weary until you bring me into*
> *the wine cellar,*
> *until your left hand is under my head and your right arm*
> *blissfully embraces me; and you kiss me with the most*
> *blissful kiss of your mouth.*
>
> WORDS OF SAINT CLAIR OF ASSISI,
> FROM *THE LETTERS TO AGNES,*
> TRANSLATED BY JOAN MUELLER

Now, dear readers, I shall switch writing styles so that you can feel for yourselves the change in voice as I move into the heart's alchemy of longing, gratitude, and rapture. Because this energy is so key to our transformation in sacred union, I encourage you to open to the experience yourselves. Within these spaces I find God so very alive, embracing, present, and real. The gap within our relationship closes; the impersonal becomes so very personal. To summarize, I have experienced time and time again how longing transports me to God, to a place within my consciousness where we share our love for one another, soul to soul, creator and created.

I long for you . . .

Will I ever reach the piece of earth or time and space
where I can lay down at your feet this longing that I
have carried throughout the history of creation?

Will I ever discover the shores of your soul, where I can
crawl on my hands and knees out of the tumulus
ocean into your arms for just one moment?

Who are you that I speak of? What are you?

Why do you haunt me so, tormenting my every waking
awareness with your ungraspable presence from the
setting of the sun until its first rays flicker at my
eyelids once again?

I see beauty in you, as I become a mirror that cannot
close its eyes to your longing to know me . . .

I love you so absolutely that the only reason my heart
beats is to know you more.

Your glory breathes me, and still I want you closer than
my breath.

O gracious and eternal love, will the gift of my life be
ever enough to lay at your feet?

Thank you, thank you for your presence in my life!

And after gratitude, the rapture . . .

How do I stand this? This torment of knowing and
not knowing you so deeply.

All I can muster is deep wild devotion as I stretch
myself out in homage to you!

Do what you will, I am yours, yours—always and
forever . . .

HEALING THE
WOUNDS OF THE HEART

In order to reach the pure states of longing and gratitude that lead to rapture and divine union, we humans must bravely face and clear any obstacles to this opening of the heart. As many of you have already discovered through years of relationships, as soon as you start getting close it's only a matter of time before the wounds begin to surface. I have noticed that the masculine and feminine polarities within us carry distinct and separate wounds of love. The feminine principle often fears abandonment, disappointment, and betrayal of her heart. The masculine principle can often experience a sense of getting trampled on, used, or losing his love from some outside force. One of his deep secret fears is of his heart breaking or being taken. It is sometimes said that a man only truly loves once and can never fully recover from his first heartbreak.

When I examine this controversial observation of the masculine I discover that the limitation placed upon him is not a hard and fast rule. When a man has developed an authentic connection with his feminine principle—with the elements of compassion, kindness, nurturing, rest, and forgiveness—then he can magnificently move on. In the past the masculine was frowned upon if he entered his grief and sorrow, even in the privacy of his own home. Men have so often been culturally conditioned to shut down these distinctly healthy feminine ways of restoring the balance within the heart. By the power of releasing grief and the anointment of applying self-love and kindness any man can cleanly move on from a broken heart.

As a woman, if you sense this wound within your man you can tenderly hold his heart space and commune with his feminine nature as you extend the presence of your holy love. It is very important work for the woman to help nurture her partner's feminine side in a delicate and nonintrusive way.

These preparatory stages of sacred union are intended to be one of the most profoundly transformative periods of your lifetime. Look at all the types of love in your life, sincerely seek to transform all relationships, feel into wild longing, gratitude, and the alchemy of divine rapture. Be willing to heal the heart so it can be a vessel of love, wisdom, and power, thereby transporting you to a sense of bliss way beyond our understanding. All this time we imagine that we are preparing for our twin soul, that we are clearing the path for him or her to enter. But in fact we are transforming the entirety of our being on Earth to reflect the true and lasting beauty of our own united soul. Every meticulous inner movement of discomfort in varying forms is used as an ally to highlight areas where a state of separation still exists.

When two people commit to this process they will experience a crucible of alchemical friction that creates the vibrational frequency required to responsibly embody the luminescence of Christ consciousness. This is sacred work.

WHAT WOULD LOVE DO?

Because we are often injured regarding our relationships and understanding of love, the question "What would love do?" can be better understood as "What would God's love do?" or "What would my soul do?" Often our injuries with love cause us to have an incomplete view of love, most often arising from the wounded child within. These injuries usually manifest themselves in either poor self-love or selfishness when dealing with others. When we ask "What would God's love do?" we are attempting to see our partner and ourselves as God sees us, and we come to understand that our feelings and our partner's feelings are of equal importance to God.

Now, because a relationship involves two people, the question "What would love do?" must be applied to both persons within the relationship. In addition, when asking this question it must be asked from two perspectives. First, what would my love of myself do? Second, what would my love for my partner do? Each person in the relationship needs to ask the same questions.

When you attempt this process with your beloved it is *crucial* that you do this when you are together and that you openly share anything that arises in the moment. Ideally you would ask these questions when experiencing conflict and misunderstanding by highlighting where you have lost your center and moved from the heart into ego—although the beauty of this exercise is so exquisite that these questions could be asked every day to align with truth and love.

Sacred Initiation

Take some quiet time with pen and paper as you feel into this process. At first do this by yourself, and then, when it feels right, do this with your partner.

AJ Miller and Mary Luck from Australia shared these questions with me a few years ago. Their work is known throughout the world as the Divine Truth Foundation and is a sincerely recommended source of profoundly clear and sincere teachings. When I asked myself these very questions I was astonished at the level of clarity and utter realization that poured through the answers. As they came to me the warmth of truth resonated throughout my body; there was no doubt, no confusion, only the silence of humility and beauty.

Now I invite you to ask yourself these questions:

What would my love for myself motivate me to do for myself?

What would my love for my partner motivate me to do for him or her?

What do I feel my partner's love for him- or herself would motivate my partner to do for him- or herself?

What do I feel my partner's love for me would motivate him or her to do for me?

Each partner asks from his or her own perspective and writes the answers.

When you are both done share your answers. Read and *feel* your responses to your partner's answers. Be honest and tell the truth about your feelings if you feel a disagreement. Share with your partner openly how the answers make you feel. Are you in agreement with the answers? Is your partner in agreement with your answers?

If any of your partner's answers to the four questions creates a sensation of inaccuracy within you, you must address this feeling immediately while still asking the question "What would love do?" For instance, you may get an inner sensation that arises with a form of communication like this:

No, my love for myself would not allow this.

No, my love for my partner would not allow this.

No, my partner's love for me would not allow this.

No, my partner's love for him- or herself would not
   allow this.

In that moment you must speak the truth, still in the spirit of "What would love do or say?" If one or both of you in the relationship is unwilling to discuss or resolve the differences, then there are problems. Over the course of time these problems, if left unaddressed, will result in the decay of the relationship.

Within these four questions and answers you have the key to unlocking the deep subconscious blocks that you may be experiencing. These questions cut straight to the truth of love, so you can see clearly where the issues lie and your own part in the avoidance or resistance to love—your part in denying your self-love. If we avoid acting, speaking, and feeling the truth of love all we are doing is denying our experience of it and sabotaging our ability to heal and grow. With the intelligence of our wounded child we imagine that we are withholding our love from our partner as a form of punishment. Yet all we are doing is withholding it from ourselves.

If one partner is unwilling to ask his or her personal set of four questions of him- or herself, there is a high likelihood that the decay of the relationship will occur. Often, many are willing to ask the questions that relate to the other person but are totally unwilling to ask the personal questions that will resolve the issues within. When both partners are willing to answer all questions, then it becomes apparent that the relationship may continue—but that will depend on the truthful answers from the questions and the required actions taken by two people attempting to live by honoring their feelings and emotions.

In the light of this truth see how you can work together to find a solution that love can stand beside.

Remember that love does not compromise. Love only knows "win/win."

I move forward with trust and consciousness.

5

GRATITUDE
The Wounds of Love

I have been apart and I have lost my way,
The archons have taken my vision.
At times, I am filled with Thee,
But often I am blind to Thy Presence,
When all I see is this world of form.
My ignorance and blindness are all I have to offer,
But these I give to Thee, holding nothing back
And in my hours of darkness,
When I am not even sure there is a Thou
Hearing my call, I still call to Thee with all my heart.
Hear the cry of my voice, clamoring from this desert,
For my soul is parched and my heart can barely stand this
    longing.

HOLY SOPHIA'S WORDS,
FROM "RITUAL OF THE BRIDAL CHAMBER,"
BY BISHOP ROSAMONDE MILLER

These are the words of the Holy Sophia, taken from the Gnostic
Mystery of the Eucharist (Ecclesia Gnostica Mysteriorum). They reveal

her inner torment as she descends to Earth in the attempt to save humankind, her children. Since discovering this prayer many years ago I have been using it when lost in my own moments of quiet despair, or when the mind has gained a powerful grip and the light of my heart has seemingly diminished.

As we step into the second chapter of the heart mysteries we come to face the wounds of love. This sacred teaching came to me during the 2009 Easter weekend after being shown an original painting of the five wounds of Christ that was once held in the Vatican vaults. This painting was so powerful that for the next forty-eight hours I was consumed with a passion that brought these insights.

For years I had been praying to understand the nature of the Crucifixion in terms of the energetic significance. I asked myself over and over why there were five wounds, not four, not six. Five represents the pentagram, Venus, and the Divine Feminine. Why was Christ wounded by Venus, by love herself?

There was no doubt in my heart that Jesus Christ was the embodiment of absolute love and that his entire being longed for us all to embody what he knew. I contemplated the passion of Christ and the events leading up to the Crucifixion and asked myself, at the deepest levels, was this path an initiation into the full sacred heart? Was this process one that we all walk, in one way or another? I eventually realized that Mary Magdalene also had to face these same tests. The five wounds lead us directly to the heart of the passion.

* First wound: betrayal
* Second wound: denial
* Third wound: judgment
* Fourth wound: separation
* Fifth wound: abandonment

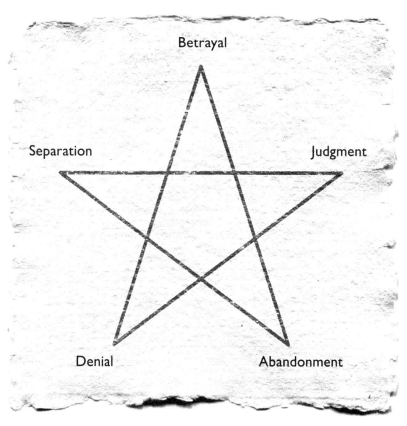

Pentagram of the Five Wounds

FACING THE WOUNDS

Before you flee in the opposite direction I am not suggesting that we all have to face the same torturous ordeal that Jesus did. However I am quietly confident that we may well have to face the same human wounds as we surrender deeper into love and one another. To love without fear is our goal and deep desire, and when we set ourselves a task of this nature many a god and demon shall appear on the horizon to hold us back.

This initiation was not limited to the sacred couple of Jesus and Mary Magdalene, for in truth every pair of beloveds who truly seek to reunify will walk the same sacred path. My research revealed indisputable evidence that historical, archetypal, and modern-day beloveds would at some point be led toward this initiation of the wounds of love. Not only that, but even those seeking to know the fullness of God's love by taking the ascetic's path—being alone and renouncing everything—must still face the very same obstacles.

This was an astonishing insight.

What we have here is a formula, a sequence of initiations that a soul has to pass through to come to know and be the love of God.

Whether we do it alone or with another in sacred union, there is no escaping the wounds of love. Do your own research, and you will be astounded at what you find. From Lemuria to ancient Egypt, from the Arthurian legends to the bloodline of Christ, from the Hindu gods to the Greek pantheon. As Sophia and the Logos, Isis and Osiris, Adam and Eve. This path of initiation is one that the whole Grail lineage, or Rose Line, must experience to fully mature and initiate the heart in order to consciously receive the love of God/Source.

The alchemical process of sacred union has never been about containing this love for your partner and yourself. It has *always* been motivated by the impulse of a deep and eternal prayer to be of the greatest service and devotion to love, in its divine meaning of agape.

As we know love does not wound, yet paradoxically these wounds do exist. Furthermore, it is only through the mystery of love that they emerge and seek refuge within our hearts from the dark abyss of being denied. How they got there in the first place no one can really know for sure. However, some modalities of wisdom can shed light on some of the possible reasons why they emerge within us when walking toward the arms of love.

My research led me toward the moment of creation, a fundamental moment in time when we lost connection with our Creator, our source of love. Whether this was part of the great plan or not doesn't really matter. What matters is that it happened, and my purpose in writing this book is to transform the deeply buried feelings that we may have about this. We can use many mind tricks to spiritually justify these feelings, but it doesn't get us anywhere. True transformation emerges when we stop running and turn to face one of humankind's greatest pains—the wound of separation. According to my innermost knowing these wounds surface within us whenever we come into contact with a deep love, because by its very nature love seeks to touch the raw scar of when it severed from itself.

The transformation of the wounds of love happens within the deepest alchemical chambers of the heart. It takes a blend of trust, faith, forgiveness, surrender, and service for one to willingly bear the process of rebuilding one's connection fully back to love/God/Source. This initiation of love becomes the process that will spearhead the full reunion of our hearts with the Source. Once this transformation happens and we reach the gateway to the ritual of sacred union, we can truly say that fear does not ever shadow our hearts.

My research for a plausible explanation for the original cause of these wounds led me toward *The Right Use of Will* books by Ceanne DeRohan, which I highly recommend. According to Ceanne's writings creation was not perfect; in fact, it was a period of trial and error. With error, as we know, comes pain. The other model of the creation story that I sometimes refer to is the Garden of Eden, which is the story of how humankind fell from grace when we took a bite of the apple (wisdom) from the Tree of Knowledge. I also take references from the *Pistis Sophia,* which gives an entirely different perspective on the root of the original cause of our separation. Yet this work also recognizes the fundamental worlds of separation based on ignorance and blindness.

My sense is that there was a moment in time when we, as humankind, were transported from an existence of paradise and beauty into a world of polarity, a sensory realm of both light and dark energies. The shock and ramifications of this can still be felt today, deep within our collective psyche. I also found these same creation stories throughout the many cultures and religions of the world. This underlines the archetypal truth that something of this nature must have happened at some point in our existence as humankind.

We can accept, then, that the wounds of love happened as a result of our original separation, real or imagined, from our creator. Thus it is by *entering* these very wounds that we get to glimpse our return home. Could this be the reason why Christ and Mary Magdalene, as well as all other beloveds that I have stumbled across, so obviously entered this process?

It has become clear. Every wound of separation holds a key to the heart. Instead of running from feelings like disappointment, embarrassment, irritation, resentment, anger, jealousy, and fear, we can choose to see that these feelings accurately teach us where we are holding back. They teach us to perk up and lean in when we feel we'd rather collapse and back away. They're like messengers that show us, with terrifying clarity, exactly where we're stuck. In the moment these kinds of feelings arise, we must choose to pay attention and realize that within our hands are the keys to freedom.

- ✳ Betrayal
- ✳ Denial
- ✳ Judgment
- ✳ Separation
- ✳ Abandonment

All these wounds are held within the mind/psyche, whereas their healing balm is discovered within the deep warmth of the all-embracing heart. Each wound is a particular frequency pattern that requires a certain touch of love from the heart, which will break open its hardened shell. For me this anointing touch has only been experienced when in the profundity of a soul-to-soul connection with God. Whenever I look back

I realize that every time I walked through a wound of love it was during an epiphany of undeniable God realization: one of those moments where I felt my heart was going to burst because I was humbled in the presence of the Creator. In all my years of spiritual initiation the great work has only ever been done when receiving a one-on-one with God! In sacred union we have to first individually carve open those true and innocent paths that lead from the purity of our heart to God's.

When we embark upon this work we have to remember that our partner will also be going through the same process. Remember with compassion that there will be numerous times when your partner will be deep within his or her process and may not be able to receive you fully in your moments of pain. During those times it would be incredibly wise to turn to God, praying to receive the anointment of divine truth and love. When you are in pain commune deeply within, in a feeling state of prayer, and ask to receive clarity as to where these wounds stem from and how to release and integrate them. Only when most of the wound has been felt and accepted into your heart for gentle tender healing is it appropriate to share with your partner. It is also important to note that sharing is indeed an important part of this process, even after the healing is complete. If you are both entered fully into the healing of the wounds of love do not keep anything hidden or unspoken. But do let God be the first point of reference in the moment that resistance or pain arises. Turn to God in prayer, asking for the truth regarding a situation and for the anointment of love.

In the silence of your feeling heart and soul, you will sense the response.

Throughout the day, I had watched Yeshua [Jesus] move among the people, filling those around him with healing and laughter. My love for him, always so alive, welled up like a fountain inside me until I had no place untouched by that love. In loving him, my love poured out to the entire world.

When Yeshua and I were alone, as if he had known my earlier thoughts, he said, "There are those who say they love me, but unless their love embraces every creature, extending from the highest to the lowest spheres, they know not love at all: For I live not only here in this form beside you, but in all of the worlds. There is no part of life in which I am not scattered. You, Miriam, truly love me, for your love knows no bounds. It touches every fragment, for it encompasses the All."

An excerpt from *The Testament of Miriam of Magdala,* edited and translated by Rosamonde Miller

The above passage exquisitely portrays how two beings live and feel when they have unified at the level of the heart. This is the true way of love, to emit a tangibly felt radiance that pours forth from two hearts that know no fear. This love touches and embraces all sentient beings in its wake.

THE ANOINTMENTS OF LOVE

The five anointments of love are the antidotes to the wounds. To the mind these healing nectars seem preposterous and almost impossible to apply in one's contracted moments of pain. However, it is precisely the use of paradox that will crack open the hardened shell of the wound—I know this by direct experience. Only the enormity of the sacred heart can contain such an implosion in these moments of seeming chaos. In order to transform, however, you must desire this shift—even more than "being right"! The wound has it's own justifications. All sense of pride must go; all egoic structures that keep you protected and in control must dissolve. When we embark upon the path of heartfelt union we must witness this resistance in ourselves and consciously choose love. We must be ultimately committed to wanting love above and beyond everything else. Despite appearing vulnerable, fragile, unprotected, defenseless, and naked, you still serve love. Your beloved in his or her wounded state may challenge you to pick up your ego and thrash out a few more stories of separation and competition. But the Lover with a capital L inwardly prays for divine grace to anoint both of your hearts.

* Trust
* Truth
* Forgiveness
* Surrender
* Service

The above five words are the same heartfelt states that every other beloved couple has entered to transform the wounds of separation.

What I am about to share is highly controversial and may cause great resistance within you, and yet I can only share what I have experienced. You can read the full story of how I moved through the wounds of love in the *Pilgrimage of Love,* my first novel. But for now I shall simply summarize.

Betrayal and Trust

When you are experiencing a sense of betrayal—even sexual infidelity—you must be willing to trust that this experience is part of your soul's greater evolution. Even this act of tremendous pain is a teaching of love. It is important to feel and honestly confess to yourself the heat of your passionate response and all the varying emotions that you will feel. In fact, this is an integral part of the transformation. When that has subsided, then apply the anointment of trust.

Release in your mind what your partner did or didn't do, come into prayer with God, ask to receive God's divine love and truth regarding the matter, and *trust* the process. The mind will want to jump back to your partner and the drama. The mind will want to remind you that you are a victim. But this is the moment of discipline and commitment.

Come to God and for a moment forget your partner, take your hot heart and fragile soul to God for transformation. If you have a truly loving and conscious partner he or she can be with you during this process, holding your hand or simply bearing witness. But please do not discuss the drama, unless it is conscious and open. Your partner will also be in a vulnerable state. When fully being with the wounds of love—whether you are receiving or instigating—one partner is not more elevated than the other. Each role must be played, and you may be required to play each part at different times.

When all betrayal dissolves, eros in its fullness and purity is revealed and can be joyfully submerged into.

Denial and Truth

When you are experiencing the urge to deny and turn away from truth, instead have faith and simply move toward it in the desire to express truth. The movement of denial, be it internal or external, is to turn away, move backward, side step, or to blatantly ignore. In this process I am suggesting you take the opposite direction. Move forward in faith, toward the contraction, to shine the light of your consciousness on what you are denying and with courage speak or act on the truth. Powerfully declare your allegiance to love *now* in this moment, despite your egoic pride. Truth rises from an inexhaustible source of love. Truth requires no proof, no evidence, no tangible reason for its being— it just is. This is the quality that can transform the heaviest and densest of wounds.

There is an old saying that goes "Tell the truth and shame the devil." This is what I am referring to when I say truth. Declare the truth of your love, declare the truth in your sacred union process, declare the truth of your integrity, have faith in your beloved's capacity to stand beside you when revealing truth, and be true to the love of your soul to become clear and free of the wounds to love. Denial of truth injures your soul—and that is a *truth*.

When all denial dissolves, philia in its fullness and purity is revealed and can be joyfully submerged into.

Judgment and Forgiveness

When receiving judgment, whether it is inner or outer, apply the healing balm of forgiveness. "What, you've got to be joking!" I hear the ego cry. I understand how impossible this seems in the moment. Trust me, I have been on the receiving as well as the instigating end of this wound and yes, it is rough sailing. However, there are no winners with these wounds because the game is not designed that way. The wounds lie within the territory of mind and are slaves to the prideful ego. They will do anything to stay alive within our thoughts, and they will produce myriad reasons for not trusting, telling the truth, forgiving, surrendering, and serving love.

Judgment carries a seductive trap. We imagine that we will die if we forgive our judgers and judgments. In a way that is a true assessment, because what forgiveness involves is bearing the unbearable. Who you *think* you are can't do it. Who you *really* are can do it. The false self—who you think you are—dies in the process. I confirm that has been my direct experience. As I have mentioned, on this path you must want love more than anything—even more than being right and even more than feeling justified.

When all judgment dissolves, storge in its fullness and purity is revealed and can be joyfully submerged into.

Separation and Surrender

Separation, that cold and icy state of numbness, happens when you lose all feeling and connection to love and your beloved. We all know this one, right? When something has been said or done that hurts us deeply instead of coming forward and confessing our wound and pain, we shut down. The tendency of separation is to withdraw just at the moment the pain comes. We immediately ice over so as not to feel more pain.

There is no attempt made to consciously address the situation, just absolute closure. In many ways we cast out our beloved in this reaction of separation. We banish him or her from our hearts and souls; we run them out of town with not a word as to the reason why. This is clearly felt by our beloved, and yet when asked what has happened and what we are feeling we tend to deny all knowledge and say "I don't know" or "Nothing."

We do know, everyone knows, but we have become so stuck in the firm belief that we are right and that it is wisest to remain protected and defended.

That's where surrender comes in.

My beloved friends, we must find a way to surrender back into our hearts, and I know it is not easy. I often find my way back to surrender by playing some incredibly emotive music and praying out loud for divine help. I ask to surrender into my heart. Sometimes I pray to the Holy Sophia, as I have faith that she too knows the enormity of the power within the wounds of ignorance. I pray to Sophia and ask her to remind me how to feel, knowing that she too became blind and lost within the deceptive realms of forgetfulness. In this process there is something about hearing my own voice crying out into the cosmos that seems to crack the shell of my own separation from love. May you find your own way back also. It is a process each of us must walk through with passion and humility, reminding ourselves of our ultimate desire for unity with love.

When all separation dissolves, agape in its fullness and purity is revealed and can be joyfully submerged into.

Abandonment and Service

Abandonment is that heavy feeling of being dropped, not included, rejected, and left. The feelings of abandonment suggest that you hide away forever and refrain from all life-sustaining activities when this incredible weight descends upon you. When Yeshua (Jesus Christ) was on the cross his last words reveal for a moment the foreboding enormity of the abandonment that came over him as he asked, "Father, why hast thou forsaken me?" These words reveal to us that the presence of the last wound was experienced just moments before his liberation. And yet at the actual moment of his death we hear him proclaim an inner shift from abandonment to the remembrance of his service to love as he says, "Father, unto your hands, I commit my spirit." That sentence tells us everything—job done!

When it comes to the initiation of abandonment I am here to remind you of your greater service to love. Like all the other wounds, abandonment draws us inward and toward a sense of empty loneliness. What I am suggesting is to move the other way, to bravely align with your oath of love, and to come forward as you proclaim your allegiance to love. Open to the experience of abandonment with a remembrance of your vows of love and service to the whole of humanity.

Remember *why* you are doing this; never forget *why* you have initiated this process. These reasons are far greater than your wounded child. If you feel that your partner has attempted to abandon you and you are committed to the sacred union process, do not accept or believe him or her. Hold firm and hold true and wait for the storm to pass. I know that you, the reader of this book, have likely played out your abandonment wounds many times in this lifetime. I know that now you are ready to choose something different.

Make your commitment to the living presence of trust, truth, forgiveness, surrender, and service to love. Recognize you have never been truly abandoned, nor will you ever be. Choose to penetrate the illusion and claim your oneness with the Source, now and forever.

When all abandonment dissolves, rapture in its fullness and purity is revealed and can be joyfully submerged into.

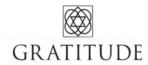

GRATITUDE

The sweet balm of gratitude allows us to open our hearts once again to God, to love, and to our soul. Feel gratitude that you have found a path where your partner and yourself can come to know and love one another without fear. Know with gratitude that there is a path that you can walk with your beloved toward the fullness of your heart and the sacredness of sexuality. This path encompasses everything; it is a journey where nothing is left out, one in which you truly do have the keys to the Kingdom of Heaven.

When you look ahead and see the potential that stretches out in front of you, you will indeed be rendered speechless with an overflowing heart.

Gratitude is also an aspect of the masculine heart. Often the masculine journey through life has been a lonely path. The old paradigm has brainwashed the man to suppress his feminine side and the expressions of his feelings. In this way he can never come to know love as deeply as his feminine counterpart. I am not saying that he does not love as deeply, but rather that his depth of feeling is often numbed and disregarded. Unlike women, men steer clear of overwhelming feelings, imagining that they might lose their minds or that they would lose control. Yet in this avoidance they are crippled and denied the freedom to know chaos, to know the essence of Shakti herself.

A woman's multidimensional range of emotional expressions allows her to more easily know God and the very nature of life, death, and rebirth. Yogi Bhajan, the last living master of kundalini yoga, would often tell me that a woman has sixteen times more emotional velocity than a man, meaning we have a much richer and wider experience. If you are a woman take some time to contemplate how it would feel to lose the majority of that field of expression and relationship to life. It can bring up an overwhelming sense of compassion and more patience with the essential differences between the masculine and feminine essences. Women, our hearts must reach out toward the men, not only for those on this journey but for all men everywhere.

One of the greatest wounds of the masculine is the fear of being rejected by the feminine. It's different from the abandonment issue for women. This rejection doesn't involve a push; it comes as a cold and icy turning away. The masculine feels that if that happens he will die. Paradoxically he also carries the fear of being consumed. There is an incredible dichotomy, a love/hate battle going on inside him. Although he knows deep inside that if the feminine did reject him he would die, he nonetheless resists the feeling of being consumed. This can relate to his mother; there is indeed death with no womb to birth into, no milk to suckle on, no love to feel, and no soft warm body to hold. Yet if his mother does not let him go at the correct developmental time, his nourishment can turn to resentment and fear of being consumed. Understanding this archetypal battle in the masculine psyche can help women hold loving space for their men.

The way for a man to penetrate these wounds is by the grace of gratitude. Many times I have witnessed men surrendering into the flow of gratitude as they were reminded of the eternal and endless love of the Holy Sophia, the feminine face of God. This grace did not come in an intellectual way; it came through me by engaging the essence of my heart and soul to reflect to them the absolute timeless truth of her love.

I feel that women now are being primed to access the Holy Sophia within themselves and to bravely speak the words from the depths of their hearts that men long to hear.

> *I have always been with you*
> *I have whispered your name in the rustle of the leaves of*
>   *autumn*
> *I have called to you with the voice of the waves of the sea*

I have watched you while I hid in the clouds
The birds have sung my messages
And I have given you echoes of my presence through all eyes
that have looked at you.
For in all creatures exists a spark of my presence
I have waited for you, my Beloved
For I have loved you and longed to give you life.

FROM "RITUAL OF THE BRIDAL CHAMBER,"
BY BISHOP ROSAMONDE MILLER

I sense that the feminine principle will be leading and cultivating this process of sacred union only until the point when the masculine heart opens. When the man gets a taste for what is possible a whole new world will open for him. After that beloveds will move forward together in the paradigm of sacred union, which they are restoring to Earth.

Sacred Initiation for Gratitude

Your work for this chapter is very simple and yet may prove to be the most difficult. I am asking you to pray out loud every day, by yourself and together with your beloved.

I invite you to listen to your own voice and the voice of your beloved. Listen for the sincerity in your voices. At first it may not be there and you may have to climb mountains of resistance and pride. This is good, as those illusionary mountains are blocks to your progress. Eventually it will filter through.

Somehow we shall establish that innocent reconnection with God/love/Source/soul in a heartfelt way. Your prayers will not come from your mind but will instead be vulnerably spoken from your innermost heart.

Here is one of my prayers, which I used when I was seeking to be cleansed from the five wounds of love.

Dear Mother Father God,

I pray to you with the sincere pure longing within my
  soul to reach and connect with you, my Creator. I
  humbly pray to receive your divine love into my soul
  as I venture into the dark pastures of my past as I
  reclaim my consciousness of where I am still holding
  the wounds of love.

Please God, please fill me with your divine truth so I
  may fully come to realize and feel where I still feel a
  sense of betrayal (denial, judgment, separation, and
  abandonment). I cannot do this without you [Mother/
  Father—your choice].

Help me to connect with my true feelings around these
  wounds so I may wash clean the error from within my
  soul, so I may authentically be able to one day truly
  connect with my soul half in the masculine/feminine
  form without carrying this injury.

Dear Mother/Father, it is my sincere prayer to become
  whole and innocent again, so I may shine forth your
  love and truth everywhere within my life.

I truly love you with my whole heart and rejoice for the
  day when I know that I am with you constantly.

Amen.

Be sure that you pray for the healing of one wound at a time. For instance, on one day you would say, "Please, God, please fill me with your divine truth so I may fully come to realize and feel where I still feel a sense of betrayal," and then on the next day you would say, "a sense of denial," and so on.

Suggestions

* Create the right environment
* Light some candles
* Play heartfelt music
* Spend some time relaxing and concentrating on the breath
* Read some poetry, perhaps Rumi, Hafiz, or Saint Clair
* Finally, speak to God, love, your soul

I pray that you begin to access a sense of your own pristine and tender longing and gratitude for all that you are and shall become.

I move forward with trust and consciousness.

6

RAPTURE
The Bridal Chamber

There exist forms of union
Higher than can ever be spoken,
Stronger than the greatest forces
With the power that is their destiny.
Those who live this are no longer separated
They are one.
Is it not necessary for those who know this to recognize one
*   another?*
Yet some do not, and they are deprived of this joy.
Those who recognize each other
Know the joy of living together in this fullness.

THE GOSPEL OF PHILIP,
TRANSLATED BY JEAN-YVES LELOUP

We have reached a stage of this heartfelt journey in which all that has been retrieved, transformed, and celebrated is now surrendered to something even greater. As we merge ever deeper into the ancient teachings of sacred union we come to a threshold known as the sacrament of the heart. Remember that the word *sacrament* means an outward and visible sign of an internal and spiritual grace. Here is a moment upon our journey where you are being invited to know truth.

As Osho, the Indian mystic, guru, and spiritual teacher, once said, "Truth can never be told, it can only be tasted."

I wholeheartedly agree. To know truth one has to feel it, live it, and become it. I believe the only way to know truth is to throw yourself into experience. What I am about to share can be seen as controversial, and it is also one of the best conversation boosters among consenting adults!

During my years of exploration into sacred union, in almost every tradition that I encountered, I would come across the notion of withholding both the orgasm and ejaculation as a central pillar of the process. At first I wasn't impressed with such an idea! Yet my yogic background at first whispered, and then blatantly shouted, that this information contained valuable wisdom. As I looked deeper into the teachings I could clearly see how a retained orgasm and ejaculation that was channeled through the spine, chakras, glands, and nadis had the power to massively open and strengthen the spiritual fire and nervous system within us. I had to tread carefully through this insight, however, as it came up against prevailing Christian beliefs that sex was bad, sinful, and certainly not spiritual.

And yet my inner wisdom whispered that there were truths woven into these esoteric sexual teachings. In the spirit of discovery I embarked upon the next stage of this journey. I gave myself a 120-day practice period, because my old kundalini yoga teacher, Yogi Bhajan, stated that to know something and to make it yours you needed to commit to a 120-day practice. I used this time to come to know for myself how much truth was within these teachings.

My invitation to everyone who walks this path is to know thyself.

This includes the initiation into the direct experience of knowing for yourselves how you respond when withholding and channeling your ejaculation and orgasm into your subtle anatomy. My strong suggestion is to fully enter into this next phase of teachings and devote at least a lunar cycle to experience this knowledge for yourself.

As we are all conscious adults it is up to you how you respond to these teachings in relation to masturbation. Personally it seems unwise to release the orgasmic energy as one could be cheating oneself from the full wisdom that could be received from the right use of will. I say if you are to do something, do it fully.

THE SACRAMENT OF THE BRIDAL CHAMBER: WHAT WAS IT?

Sixty years ago a group of ancient texts called the Nag Hammadi codices were discovered in an urn in Upper Egypt. These ancient texts have sparked some fascinating debates about Christianity's central mystery. One of the most intriguing candidates for that mystery is the sacrament of the bridal chamber. It is described specifically in the Gospel of Philip as the means to attain Christhood. It is also alluded to in the Exegesis on the Soul and, apparently, in the Gospel of Thomas. For those raised on the traditional assumptions that Jesus was celibate and sex has a sinful element, the very suggestion that he practiced the sacrament of the bridal chamber as a path to Christhood can be both startling and tantalizing.

Yet these ancient manuscripts suggest that it is possible that Jesus taught a mystery about the union of male and female. Was the sacrament of the bridal chamber purely allegorical, or did it directly refer to a physical union? If it involved the sexual union of lovers:

* Was it a fertility rite, as portrayed in *The Da Vinci Code*?
* Was it a rite for the conception of spiritually advanced offspring

as suggested by Jean-Yves Leloup in a recent translation of the Gospel of Philip?

* Was it a means of giving birth to the Christ within, two by two, employing controlled intercourse?

For years scholars interpreted the sacrament of the bridal chamber as an allegorical union, despite the rather explicit references to intercourse in the Nag Hammadi texts. Apparently unable to imagine Jesus engaged in sexual intimacy, most translated the words implying sexual union as "marriage," and the Exegesis on the Soul was read strictly as a metaphorical account of union between the bridegroom (Jesus) and the fallen soul of (wo)man. This interpretation is in line with official Christian dogma.

Yet the actual language in the Nag Hammadi texts urges us to remove our canonical spectacles. In doing so we must consider the possibility that the church authorities mistakenly—or on purpose—narrowed the initial concept of sacred union to an allegorical tale. Following this original mistake or deception the church has interpreted new historical evidence accordingly ever since. Now observers are daring to explore the possibility that the Gospel of Philip means what it appears to say: *Intercourse, correctly performed, is an essential sacrament, and ordinary sex has unsuspected perils with spiritual implications.*

French Orthodox theologian Jean-Yves Leloup has a different interpretation of the sacrament of the bridal chamber. He points out that the Gospel of Philip envisions a "sacred embrace," which is a sexual union based not on lust but rather on the spiritual blending of man and woman.

Other observers, Cambridge scholar Mary Sharpe among them, agree that the sacrament of the bridal chamber calls for the sexual union of soul mates but not for the purpose of producing physical offspring. This reminds us that the Gospel of Thomas makes clear that better procreation was not Jesus's objective.

The gnostic goal appears to be an Immaculate Conception result-ing from a "pure embrace," or the "holy of holies," both of which refer to mindful intercourse that reunites male and female. This conception leads to the coveted second birth, that of the Christ within, and it rep-resents a return to humankind's nondual wholeness, the true awakened state in which God created us.

* We are reborn by the Christ two by two. In his breath we experi-ence a new embrace; we are no longer in duality but in unity.
* All will be clothed in light when they enter into the mystery of the sacred embrace.

What is the bridal chamber then, if not the place of trust and con-sciousness in the embrace? It is an icon of union beyond all forms of possession; here is where the veil is torn from top to bottom; here is where some arise and awaken. This sacred embrace offers us a return to the Edenic state. It offers a return to the time in consciousness when Adam and Eve had not yet been driven apart by the effects of physi-cal procreation, emotional alienation, and projections that produced dualistic perception and the birth/death cycle. As the Gospel of Philip explains:

> If woman had not been separated from man, she would not die with man. Her separation was at the origin of death. Christ comes again to heal this wound, to rediscover the lost unity, to enliven those who kill themselves in separation, reviving them in union.
>
> When Eve was in Adam, there was no death; when she was sepa-rated from him, death came. If she enters back into him, and he accepts her, there will be no more death. Jesus came to the place of separation so as to reunite all that had been separated in God.
>
> THE GOSPEL OF PHILIP,
> TRANSLATED BY JEAN-YVES LELOUP

What, exactly, is this sacred embrace that unites all that had been separated? Various texts of the Nag Hammadi collection suggest that it is physical, yet controlled, intercourse; that it is union without orgasm but with a deep, psychic merging. The embrace that incarnates the hidden union is not only a reality of the flesh, for there is also a deep mystical silence in this embrace. It does not arise from impulse or desire; it is an act of will. According to the Gospel of Thomas this spiritual reunion of male and female is the way in which we return to the Kingdom of Heaven and regain our primordial power and wholeness.

Jesus said to them, "The Kingdom will come when the two are one, and the outside as the inside, and the male with the female neither as male nor female" (Gospel of Thomas).

The Gospel of Thomas continues, "If someone experiences Trust and Consciousness in the heart of the embrace, they become a child of light. If someone does not receive these, it is because they remain attached to what they know; when they cease to be attached, they will be able to receive them."

What is required here is a huge letting go of the mind, a letting go of all that we think we know. In order to proceed with this journey one is required to sincerely move forward with the pure contents of one's heart—love, truth, and humility.

Intriguingly the Gnostic gospels are not the only sources from the past that refer to a sacred physical union between male and female toward a spiritual end loftier than physical procreation. The same concept of "going beyond our obsession with seeds and eggs" to reach a state of transcendent wholeness appears in Lao-tzu's ancient Hua Hu Ching. He recommends controlled intercourse, or "angelic dual cultivation," in which conventional orgasm is avoided in favor of the opportunity for a man and woman to mutually transform and uplift each other into the realm of bliss and wholeness. The key is a form of intercourse led by spirit rather than the sexual organs. This practice can give birth to something immortal, which refines gross, heavy energy into divine light. By contrast, during ordinary intercourse accumulated energy is discharged, and the subtle energies are dissipated and disordered in a great backward leap.

Alice Bunker Stockham, M.D., in her book *Karezza, Ethics of Marriage,* also suggests the possibility of nonphysical "offspring" being born of the sacred union of male and female. Stockham reports that there are deeper purposes and meanings to the reproductive faculties and functions than are generally understood. In the physical union of male and female there may be a soul communion of great power.

Men and women practicing *karezza*—gentle, conscious lovemaking without conventional orgasm—attest that their very souls in union take on a procreating power and that it seems to have an impregnating force. This force hugely transcends any ordinary thought force in its power and intelligence.

Stockham points out that the resulting progeny—in the form of great art, new inventions, and healing powers—can do much to improve the world, even apart from the spiritual gains from enhanced individual soul growth. In comparison, she notes the following: "The ordinary hasty spasmodic method of cohabitation is deleterious both physically and spiritually, and is frequently a cause of estrangement and separation."

There is recent neuroscience that supports the wisdom of learning to make love with controlled intercourse. Sex without conventional orgasm promotes inner equilibrium and more stable bonding because it mitigates the high/low cycle of dopamine, which is the driving neurochemical force behind sexual desire and addictions. This high/low cycle, which accompanies fertilization-driven sex, does indeed separate mates and poison unions. During the low part of the cycle lovers tend to pull away from each other or experience emotional friction as they project onto each other the unwelcome effects of natural, biologically driven neurochemical changes. This often creates a baffling attraction/repulsion dynamic in intimate relationships.

Interestingly, the Gospel of Philip specifically mentions that those who are no longer enslaved by the world rise above attraction and repulsion. To do so, however, they must receive a power that is both masculine and feminine in the bridal chamber.

Could the sages mentioned above be pointing to the same mystery as the sacrament of the bridal chamber? Is it possible that sacred sexual union, based upon controlled intercourse, is indeed a path to heightened spiritual awareness? Can fertilization-driven sex be preventing the sexes from rediscovering their innate nondual perception? Did those early Catholics succeed in burying the central mystery of Christianity for most of the past two thousand years when they condemned the gnostic point of view? Certainly the Nag Hammadi discoveries, with their intriguing descriptions of the sacrament of the bridal chamber and their parallels to other wisdoms of the past, raise these possibilities. Perhaps the only way to discover the truth is to attempt to re-create the experience of the sacrament of the bridal chamber for ourselves.

> Seek the experience of the pure embrace for it has great power.
>
> THE GOSPEL OF PHILIP,
> TRANSLATED BY JEAN-YVES LELOUP

THE ORGASMIC HEART

"What, I thought you said no orgasms?"

As we move ever deeper into the merging and melding of our hearts it is important for us to broaden any limited concepts and ideas that we may have regarding the potentiality of our energetic system. In fact, our energy system is capable of multiple orgasms, and there are many types of orgasm that a human being can experience!

These are groundbreaking ideas, yet you wouldn't be reading this book if you weren't ready to seed a new paradigm—with a new kind of orgasm!

Not only are all types of orgasm profoundly powerful ways of releasing the arrow of our creative and evolutionary intentions, but they are also a means of receiving copious amounts of light into our subtle anatomy. When I speak of subtle anatomy I refer mostly to the endocrine, nervous, meridian, and chakra systems, which bridge the seen and unseen parts of yourself. It is during the experience of sexual orgasm that one has the potential to use this bridge and gain access into myriad multidimensional realities and realms of experience. This depends entirely on the state of one's consciousness during the sexual act. It is precisely the same when it comes to other forms of orgasm. Your intention and frequency of consciousness is the key that shall turn the lock.

There are four bodies that have the capability of entering into an orgasmic state. They are:

* Khat (physical body)
* Ka (spirit body)
* Ab (heart body)
* Ba (soul body)

The reason we are looking at four instead of the three found in alchemy is that the ka body orgasm is one that we can all recognize as the rush of shivers and tingles that flow through our spine causing goose bumps and a heightened sense of expansion. I often refer to the ka body orgasm as an internal recognition that truth has just been spoken or received in some way. It manifests as a rush of shakti life force radiating through the ka body, bringing our attention to the present moment. I understand that the ka body orgasm is a method that our soul uses to say, "Yes, this is true for you!"

We shall be exploring the ten light bodies during the third stage of this journey, as the wisdom of the subtle anatomy rightfully belongs in the consciousness aspects of these teachings. When you research the light bodies you may discover that some mystery schools have a difference of opinion regarding the actual number of light bodies that are assigned to a human being. I shall be referring to the ancient Egyptian wisdom that speaks of a system of ten bodies. This system ties in beautifully with the ten *sephiroth* (spheres) in the Tree of Life. Each sephiroth is a dimensional space that the soul has to pass through in order to incarnate. As we pass through the ten dimensions of the Tree of Life we create ten bodies that are attuned to the vibrational frequency of that existential reality. These gossamer thin garments of light get progressively denser the closer we get to Malkuth (meaning "kingdom," relating to Earth or matter) and the creation of the physical body.

The heart, soul, and spirit orgasms are generated purely by the intent to receive such an experience. Energy follows thought. These energetic orgasms rely little on sexual energy as they are generated through the rapturous expansion of both life force (shakti/light) and surrender/devotion (bhakti/love). It is important to know that an energetic orgasm is where sexuality and spirituality come together and merge. The more I explored this theory, using both my masculine thirst for understanding and my feminine hunger for experience, the more enlightening these new realties became.

I came to understand that these orgasms encompass different expressions and movements of energy. There is a clear and repeatable coherence to them, which confirmed that this is something we can all experience if we are willing to expand our former limitations. For instance, the heart orgasm feels like a movement of extension, the soul orgasm is a feeling of resonating, and the spirit body, or ka, orgasm is one of expansion. As we venture in to new territories these energy orgasms will act as a catalyst to activate and strengthen our subtle infrastructure. When we orgasm in these new ways we shall start to bring in different frequencies of energy from other dimensions that will actually manifest physical changes, not only within our own bodies but all around us. Those who have been initiated will have the ability to work profoundly with the four elements of nature—earth, air, fire, and water.

All four orgasms are intrinsically linked to the four elements: the sexual orgasm is related to earth, the heart to water, the spirit to fire, and the soul to air. When all four orgasms can be generated the body will start humming and vibrating at a profoundly higher octave. As this happens, the energetic experience begins to "breathe you."

Khat (Material) Body Orgasm

The very substance that generates a physical body orgasm is *sekhem,* the fiery passions of both shakti and bhakti, fueled by the urge to merge. We all know how a physical body orgasm happens so I don't need to go into too much detail here. However, I will say this—when you make love as daughter, sister, mother, and wife, and son, brother, father, and husband in the fullness of love you will experience an orgasm beyond your known experiences.

Ka (Spirit) Body Orgasm

The energetic sensory apparatus required to experience an orgasm within the spirit body can be used through the powerful use of pranayama, special breathing practices done while concentrating on the first and second chakras. As a result of practicing kundalini yoga my frequency of ka body orgasms increased tenfold. In addition, by using the daily application of the *mula bhanda*—the root lock/pelvic floor contractions—I was able to awaken the once dormant energies of my first and second chakras and pulse them up through my spine to nourish my entire subtle anatomy. I know without any doubt that kundalini yoga carved open myriad intricate pathways within my internal energy system. This yoga can be explored with a kundalini teacher if you so desire.

Ab (Heart) Body Orgasm

The very substance that generates a heart body orgasm is love, the agape of unconditional love. It is felt as a rush of grace birthed within us in innocence as a result of transforming the wounds of love. I speak of the *ab* body orgasm here because it is an effect of the *ba* body orgasm. One cannot have a ba body orgasm without the heart overflowing in pure love. The ab body orgasm is a direct result of rapture felt in the soul.

However, one can experience an ab body orgasm by itself simply through the heightened sensitivity of generating a tremendous amount of natural love. The human heart gives and receives natural love, whereas the soul has the ability only to receive divine love from God. Many times with my beloved I have gazed into his eyes or lain in his arms, and I have become intoxicated by love, losing all orientation and coordination. This feeling of being taken by love and entering a completely surrendered state is the ab body orgasm—the moan and ecstasy of the heart.

Ba (Soul) Body Orgasm

The soul body orgasm is one of atonement. To atone means to make amends with God, to wipe clean our sin and error. When we break down the word into three alchemical pieces, we discover "at-one-ment," which takes on a whole different meaning and yet by its very nature also includes the biblical understanding. Atonement happens through a sincere and pure prayer to receive God.

Because God is an entity—an entity that *longs* to have a personal relationship with every single one of her children, and an entity that can infuse his divine love into your soul—the human heart contains natural love, a love that can be both given and received. Yet it is within the soul where we receive divine love from God. When we make a prayer to sincerely and purely come to know God he/she responds with a powerful energetic downpouring of love. We need only ask to receive—and we ask by connecting with our soul (ba) and moving it within our consciousness to connect and touch with God's soul. Yes, God has a soul.

When that happens the soul body orgasm ignites. It feels like a simultaneous explosion and implosion, an overwhelming rush of longing and gratitude that gives way to rapture, the feeling of being lifted and transported out of oneself by a divine power.

THE MEANING OF RAPTURE

Being lifted up and transported into the realms of divinity, we can know rapture as the second coming of Christ. Rapture is the essential energy of how the Christ penetrates us. Christ and the Logos are the same being, the same frequency. Remember that God sent forth the Logos, the Christ, to find Sophia, or Mary Magdalene. Rapture is also the key emotional signature that the Logos uses to reveal, touch, and merge with Sophia. Each of us, male or female, carries within a fragment of the eternal essence of the Holy Sophia. Only by opening ourselves to feel the exquisite states of rapture can the Logos eventually complete his devout longing: to find, retrieve, and to love once again his beloved Sophia through us.

Let me repeat again that this *love* is a being, an entity. This is precisely what Rumi and countless other Sufi poets tell us. They call God the beloved and the friend. In the gnostic tradition it is called the Logos.

Love is not an emotion, it is a being. It is alive. It is what created you, and it is what you are. It wants to know you, and it yearns for you to receive it deep within your heart and soul.

The Highest God, in His love for His own feminine self, sends forth into the world of matter a redeemer, a reflection of his own self, whom we call The Logos, who restores the Sophia's sight and reunites with Her. In their reunion, the lost sparks of humanity can also be made whole and with Her, be reunited with the Most High.

THE GNOSTIC BIBLE: THE PISTIS SOPHIA UNVEILED,
TRANSLATED BY SAMAEL AUN WEOR

We carry within us the alive spark of Sophia, who longs to be reunited with the Logos. When we come together to sincerely pray with a pure intent to receive the fullness of God's love, she responds. The Logos comes forth into the world of matter, right where we are, carrying within him the eternal and infinite magnetic longing of God to become *whole* through us.

Let that statement sit within you for a while.

LONGING PLUS GRATITUDE
EQUALS RAPTURE

We are all profoundly different, and beautifully so. Inevitably there will be some things that touch you deeply while others won't even penetrate the surface of the skin. Your task as beloveds is to discover what elements and sensory stimulation move you both. For my beloved and myself it is music, light, and beauty. We know that time spent in nature, appreciating the most glorious folds and curves of the land, and time at the end of a day listening to profoundly soulful music by candlelight are the ingredients needed to bring forth the current of rapture between us.

Bathing in the energies of all those beautiful experiences we will begin to speak about what we long for and how longing feels inside us. As we begin this conversation we literally catch fire from one another. His longing ignites my own, and vice versa. The more we speak about it, the more aroused the energies of longing become. Our conversation stumbles as we hopelessly attempt to scramble for the words to wrap around the mystical states that we are entering.

Longing naturally pours into gratitude. It *must* overflow and permeate into gratitude. By building and expanding the states of longing you will realize that what you yearn for the most already exists within the deepest spaces of your longing. Within the silent, still point of this realization one becomes acutely aware of the total dissolution of self. In that moment you have become both lost and found in the obliteration of individuality. When that happens rapture explodes through your consciousness on the very next inhale.

In that moment all that we can do is fumble for one another's hands using our fingers to transmit the word *yes* through a squeeze of togetherness.

Sacred Initiation for Rapture

Your sacred initiation is to open to these spaces of total dissolution of self, both alone and together. If you are choosing to experiment the withholding of orgasm, it is my suggestion to give this practice a month at the very least to experience for yourselves its benefits. For a full immersion you could use the whole of the three-month period for the wisdom aspect of the flame to truly know yourself as you move through the preparation of the soul union process. Whichever you choose, be sure to know that by withholding your orgasm (both partners), you will intensify the more soulful emotions of this unbridled experience that fully uses the energies of the sex, heart, and soul.

Your intention is to open, open deeper, and open even deeper still. Using your breath and sensory stimulus begin to enter the great abyss that contains the mysteries of your own heart. For some people, however, the feelings of longing are often feared as they sense they could become overwhelmed with emotion, while others cannot even identify what they could long for. Use your breath to focus on your intention, and work through these fears and uncertainties.

Here's a clue for those who are struggling to open this space: home. The unbearable yearning to return home—and the way home is found through the heart.

I move forward with trust and consciousness.

PART THREE

Soul Consciousness

The Third Trimester

To feel abandoned is to deny the intimacy of your present surroundings.

DAVID WHYTE, "EVERYTHING IS WAITING FOR YOU"

7
KNOW THYSELF

There are love "stories,"
and there is only obliteration into love.

You've been walking the ocean's edge,
holding up your robes to keep them dry.
You must dive naked under and deeper,
a thousand times!

Let the cords of your robe be untied.
Shiver in this new love beyond all above and below.
I have no more words.
Let our souls speak with the silent articulation of a face.

RUMI

In Greek mythology Delphi was the site of the Pythia Delphic oracle, the most important oracle in the classical Greek world. Delphi was also a major site for the worship of the god Apollo after he slew the python, a dragon who lived there and protected the navel of Earth. Upon entering the threshold of Delphi one would be asked to kneel before the words *gnothi seauton*, "know thyself," which were carved upon the lin-

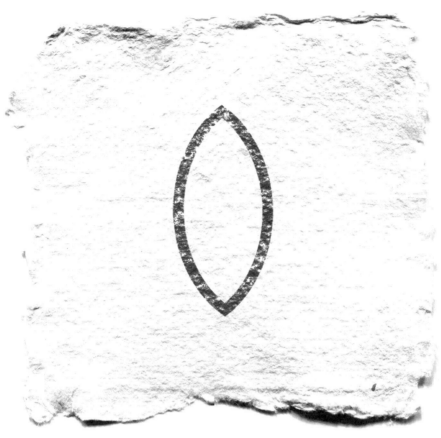

Flame

tel separating the outside from the inside, the seen from the unseen, and the ignorant from the sacred. To converse with the priestesses, the *pythia,* one had to be prepared.

There really was no other way to enter the dominion of the pythia except by those words. It is precisely by these same words that one enters sacred union. Until one knows oneself the doors of this mystical union will not open.

This chapter brings us toward the threshold of soul union, the knowledge and experience of merging consciousness. However, before we can enter we must pass the guardian who fiercely guards this third and final stage of preparation for sacred union. Here is the last test of our caliber, the test of intent and truth regarding our soul essence. As beloveds, if we are not soul halves we will not be able to pass this stage. The dragon at this gateway weeds out the weak from the strong, the false from the true, and the impostor from the rightful one. The enormity of the words *know thyself* hovers above us, inviting us to kneel as we approach the completing element of the three-fold flame—the flame of wisdom and consciousness. Herein arises the invitation to merge the totality of our consciousness with the beloved, leaving no stone unturned, no secret chamber for our own contemplations and fantasies. We are asked to fully throw open the doors to our inner world and lovingly reveal how we operate within the spaces and dimensions of our inner life.

The inner freedom that the masculine finds within his solitary consciousness often functions as a safe haven from the outside world and its many demands. This has to be gently acknowledged by the feminine as we approach the doorway to conscious union. A man's inner world is often a closely guarded aspect of himself, kept privately within his secret chambers. A woman needs to understand that this part of the journey can be as challenging for him as approaching the sexual gates is for her.

> Consciousness is where the masculine has been hiding
> and not sharing.

> Sexuality is where the feminine has been hiding
> and not sharing.

There needs to be a delicate honoring of this energetic configuration that we have used to avoid deep intimacy and stay safe from one another. Yet at the same time we can vow to stay true to the courageous journey that we have undertaken. We can meet one another with the fullness of our sexuality and consciousness within the alchemical chambers of the heart.

My invitation is for you to open as deeply as you did with your sexuality and heart—to share your consciousness with as much joy and longing as you shared your heart and sex. Who among you is warmly ready to allow the other to investigate your morals, values, and faith, as they would your passions, heartfelt dreams, sexual pleasure, and bodily longing?

You may be surprised to discover just how closed we are to such an idea. What I have seen over the years of working with individuals and couples is that this third aspect of the threefold flame can present quite a sizable challenge. It seems that our inner world is an area where we cling to our individuality and refuse to reveal or share it. This becomes the last stronghold for the separate ego identity to hide. Quite often it will even stage a self-sabotaging drama.

In my vision of working with this flame of wisdom and consciousness I sense that we would experience a higher success rate if we approach this work as individuals first, just as we did with the flames of power and love. This way we become sincerely honest with ourselves, venturing within the dimensional spaces inside to create the foundation stone for a highly evolved way of relating. Know thyself. These words encapsulate this third and final stage of preparation work before we enter the sacred union process.

Know thyself can be received as an invitation to shine the light of our consciousness into all our internal affairs, even the ones that make us squirm when we realize the real truth of what we get up to.

When we know ourselves unflinchingly we can come to know the other in a far deeper way. True openness is not only a way of vulnerably expressing and sharing who you are but also a means to receive who the other is. Because your two selves and souls are on a journey to merge back into one, the words *know thyself* apply to you both individually and as one. Remember once again the three essential keys for this journey:

Trust (sexuality)

Humility (heart)

Consciousness (wisdom)

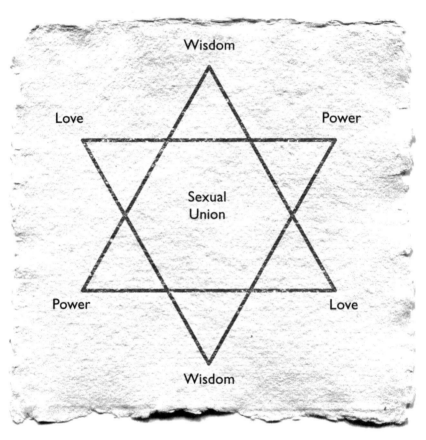

Star of David, Sexual Union and the Threefold Flame

CONSCIOUS COMMUNICATION

Knowing thyself is a threefold affair. One of the essential things to practice is conscious communication. This means total transparency with yourself and the other. Telling the complete truth until you reach the end point of unveiling your real motivations and the fueling emotions behind them. At first this may not be an easy or comfortable process, but it is absolutely necessary and vital for high-vibration relating. It is also deeply, deeply rewarding.

In my opinion conscious communication has to be first and foremost on your list of daily priorities. There is truly only one way this reunification process is going to reach its ultimate fruition, and that is by keeping the communication alive. If you are not totally clear, both you and your beloved will feel it. If left unchecked these unspoken aspects of self will attach themselves to the unhealed fears in your partner until they find an unhealthy way to be expressed.

Every relationship must have a foundation of communication. When communication is not present or breaks down, what happens? A loss of intimacy, a sense of disconnection: feelings of anger, sadness, or perhaps even resentment and power struggles. If the breakdown continues it may spell the demise of the relationship.

The First Part of Conscious Communication: Regular Practice

Like any skill, communication takes practice. If we can practice good communication skills when we are feeling connected and happy, those same skills will serve us beautifully when we need them most.

When you are with your beloved take time several nights each week to learn and implement communication practices that deepen your relationship. I have found that some of the simplest and shortest practices are the most powerful. Here are some helpful steps.

1. Create the time. If you both work at home agree to stop your work, turn off your phones, and shut down your computers at 5 p.m. on specific nights of the week. It is wise to give this sacred time your priority, maybe even set aside up to four nights a week, and reserve the other three nights for your individual needs and desires.

2. Come into presence with one another. Sit across from each other, make eye contact, and breathe. As you come into the present moment leave the day behind.

3. Choose a simple practice and follow the format of the practice. Some take only a few minutes and others may take longer. This may be a simple meditation, gazing at a candle that represents truth and love, or listening to some music that brings you both into the truth of your being.

4. Once the practice is complete take turns to speak about how you feel in general and if anything is on your mind. It is important to set aside equal amounts of time for each partner to begin speaking first while the other one simply listens. My beloved and I usually set aside fifteen minutes for each person, and then another fifteen minutes to discuss, totalling forty-five minutes. Beyond that you will start to lose the attention of the other. The most powerful work can be done in short and focused sittings. Sometimes discussion is not even needed. It is healing to simply be allowed the space to speak with the full attention of the other. This can create a profound healing and intimacy.

5. Afterward relax with each other for the rest of your evening together. Personally I cannot speak enough praises for the simple cuddle. There is nothing I relish more than simply lying together on the sofa wrapped in one another's arms, listening to music as we spaciously observe the setting sun disappear beneath the landscape.

The Second Part of Conscious Communication: Divine Truth

The second part of conscious communication is prayer. When we pray to receive the divine truth about a circumstance or problematic situation and that prayer is both sincere and pure, we shall receive the truth. Usually there is an internal sensation of energy felt within our bodies as an emotional charge. With practice and awareness this translates into an instant knowing of what is true and what is false. Some of us may be given an image with words that are sensed rather than heard. Our role is to receive the response from the prayer rather than to question its validity. If we are unclear we can ask again for further clarity and precise knowing. God will do all that he/she can so that the truth emerges into you. The problem with humankind is that often we don't like the truth so instead we turn away and tell ourselves that it can't be right.

With both prayer and insightful self-inquiry, ask and you shall receive. Trust your first impressions, catch them in your awareness, and *feel* your way into your initial discoveries so that you continue to drop ever deeper into the true motivational force and causal emotion. Stay with the process to receive full understanding.

■ Divine Truth Questions

Here are some profoundly insightful questions for you to take into prayer or self-inquiry. To share these aspects of self with your beloved would not only powerfully contribute toward the building of intimacy but also give voice to the soulful realms of your existence.

Am I living my truth?

Am I expressing my truth?

Am I living and expressing God's truth?

Am I completely truthful with myself? If not, why not?

What blocks do I have to living in truth?

What addictions do I have, both physically and emotionally?

Which relationships challenge me the most to be living and
   expressing in truth? Why?

Were my parents truthful with me?

Could I be truthful with my parents?

In the past was it safer for me to lie or omit truth?

Am I truthful with my parents now?

What scares me about truth?

What emotions are in my soul about truth?

What is the truth of how I am feeling now?

What is the truth of how God sees me?

What are my desires around truth?

To grow in truth, what's my next step?

✺ The Third Part of Conscious Communication: Emotional Clearing

There are eternal and constant laws in the universe one of which is the law of attraction. A soul that is in a poor condition will generally attract pain and suffering to itself. The pain can be physical, which is usually the result of the active denial of inner emotions, or the pain can be purely emotional. Generally many of us have a large amount of fear when dealing with our internal emotions, and so we would rather not. Because of this fear it can take an even greater amount of physical and emotional pain to actually make us finally willing to face our own internal truth.

All physical and emotional suffering is the result of "missing the mark of love," which is the true meaning of sin. It matters little whether that sin is of our own making or the result of the sins of our parents, environment, or culture. It comes upon our soul, and as a subsequent effect, it imprints upon our spiritual and physical bodies. The effects of all sin can be removed from within us, no matter what or who the cause, depending on how deeply we desire to enter a loving personal relationship with our Creator. His divine love has a purifying effect on our soul, which, in turn, affects the condition of our spiritual and physical bodies. When, with the help of the Divine, we love ourselves back to wholeness, we no longer experience suffering.

Our Creator created our body as a perfect system to measure pain, and pain is always an indicator that something is wrong within. Physical pain is a response provided for the protection of our material body and emotional pain for the protection of our spiritual bodies. For example, if we put our hand on a hot stove we will quickly feel the pain of a burn, and this causes us to respond in a way that protects our hand from being burned to a cinder and totally damaged. So pain is a protection for our physical body and a reminder that placing our body in the path of fire will damage it. This causes us to exercise care in situations that may cause this pain.

In a similar way emotional pain is a reminder that if we continue a course of action that is in disharmony with our own creation we will continue to bear its consequences. For example, if I continue to express my anger with everyone who walks into my path, eventually I will be left completely alone or in the company of other angry people, because no one who is peaceful will value my company. I am continuing to sin and my soul's condition continues to degrade. I must find a way to release my anger and connect to my sadness. I must do this in a way that does not harm others, myself, or any of God's living creation.

Taking the emotional example further, if I choose to not release the sadness that causes my anger and if I then choose to continue to suppress the anger and sadness, eventually I will become depressed and I will be so unhappy that I will feel that life is not worth living. However, once I connect with my sadness and realize the truth about it I can finally release it. If I talk to my God about it the operation of his/her love will help me overcome the sadness completely so that its cause will be transmuted and healed. As a result of the cause being removed I will not be able to get angry in the same unconscious way, and I will not become depressed from suppressing all that anger and blame.

We can see from the example above that my emotional pain is an indicator that I have emotions, beliefs, practices, thoughts, words, or actions that are in disharmony with God's laws. In order to no longer experience emotional pain I must choose to see and release the soul-based causes of the emotional pain. In other words I must choose to change and grow.

It is also important to know that we can find ourselves in an environment that is in disharmony with God's laws, and then we must choose to leave that environment if we are to tend to the full bloom of our soul in this incarnation.

■ Some Practical Advice

One of the greatest causes of stagnation is our own refusal to humbly accept our true emotional and spiritual condition and, upon accepting it, to then choose to do the work to change that condition. As long as we desire to retain false mental concepts of ourselves and project to others a false impression of who we really are, it will be impossible for us to merge into the fullness of the soul reunification process. Why? Because it requires God's divine love to do so, and if we are withholding the truth of our soul condition, we will hinder our ability to receive God's love. Remember at the beginning of this book I said that it takes three elements to enter sacred union—the feminine, the masculine, and God? Well once we have done the groundwork in healing our sexuality we need the enormity of God's love to continue on. It is only with God's unconditional love that we will experience the opening and cleansing of our soul light. God is the third element without which this process will just lead to yet another normal relationship in which two people stay perfectly individual and self-sufficient. With the third element consciously evoked the full alchemy of sacred union is complete, and what was once separate is fully reunited.

So how do we go about determining who we really are? Do we even really want to know who we really are? Surely the best thing for us to decide is to be completely open and honest with ourselves, others, and especially our Creator about our own true emotional and spiritual condition.

Below are a series of questions that will help us come to terms with the truth of our emotional condition. Please answer these questions as truthfully and openly as you are able, especially if you desire to move beyond the condition of stagnation. These are the first questions one must address to begin to open the soul to receive God's love.

My advice is to ask these questions on a daily basis.

1. What events are currently happening in my life that demonstrate I am out of harmony with divine love, and how have I attracted these events to my life?
2. What emotions within me are triggered by these events, and are those emotions in harmony with truth and love?
3. Do I feel any emotional or physical pain? If so, what reasons within my beliefs, emotions, desires, or passions could there be for my experiencing this pain?
4. How do I portray myself to others, and am I being emotionally truthful and open?
5. Am I still doing things that God or a celestial angel would not do?
6. How do I really feel inside, and what tools am I using to deny my feelings?
7. Have all my actions been moral and ethical? If not, what is the emotional cause for my being immoral or unethical?
8. Do I feel comfortable with all people in all circumstances? If not, why not?
9. Do I feel comfortable when I am around my parents, and am I being myself?
10. Am I completely myself when I am with my partner?

Again spend some time alone with these questions consulting with God for further clarification. Then share with your beloved to open the doors wider still for the soul union process.

THE THREE PROMISES

The deeper we go the easier it becomes to unearth these profoundly rich truths about ourselves. At first this muscle may be a little stiff and painful to use, but over time it will become limber and deliciously toned. We are so deep and unexplored it's incredible and fun to discover the treasure hiding in our consciousness. At times this exploration can appear totally unglamorous and feel darn right ugly. But as we now know with all sacred union work these feelings simply act as guardians who stand at the threshold of yet another unprecedented breakthrough. They roar fiercely at us, "You want truth? Oh really—well how much are you willing to pay?"

Do you know what that price is? It's a tenderly warm blend of honesty, humility, and vulnerability. When two people commit to this there can be no limitations placed upon them. The whole world opens up as God's love and light pour forth into every particle of their existence.

Sacred Initiation

Let us now take the next initiation known as the three promises. My suggestion is that this work be done on a new moon to capture the energy of new beginnings. This is a practice that you do alone.

As you work through these three promises by yourself, write down your answers and contemplations into your journal. These jewels have been buried deeply in your unconsciousness for eons and now they are coming up into the light. Place your writing underneath your pillow on the night of the new moon as you fall asleep. Intend to soak up the energy of your words into your sexuality, heart, and soul—the threefold flame of your existence. Hold the energy in these three sacred chambers and daily refresh your memory of these promises as they become activated through the cycle of the moon.

The promises were made at the dawn of time and each of them is sacred.

* The first promise is to God, your Mother and Father. It represents your most divine destiny and purpose, what you have come to accomplish in the image of your Creators. It is the reason for your incarnation, the purest intention of your soul. This promise is found within your wisdom flame and consciousness.
* The second promise is to your soul half and the soul family within which you were created and that you will belong to through eternity. It represents your relationship to each of the 144 souls in your family—how you have agreed to assist them in their mission and they in yours. This promise is found within your love flame and heart.
* The third promise is to yourself. It represents how you desire to learn and grow and love within the context of incarnation. This promise is found within your flame of power and your sexuality.

Align yourself with the promises you have made for they are sacred above all else. Remember them and cherish them, and you will know the greatest joy available to humankind. Do nothing that you know to be against your sacred promises, because an error toward them is an error in your soul.

The ancient scriptures tell us that wherever the practices of sacred union take place the soil becomes fertile and the land flourishes as a tribute to the sanctity of the trust and consciousness that is inevitably created.

I move forward with trust and consciousness.

8

BODIES OF LIGHT

After the day of rest, Sophia sent her daughter Zoe, being called Eve, as an instructor, in order that she might make Adam, who had no soul, arise so that those whom he should engender might become containers of light. When Eve saw her male counterpart prostrate, she had pity upon him, and she said, "Adam! Become alive! Arise upon the earth!" Immediately her word became accomplished fact. For Adam, having arisen, suddenly opened his eyes. When he saw her, he said, "You shall be called 'Mother of the Living.' For it is you who have given me life."

"ON THE ORIGIN OF THE WORLD," FROM *THE NAG HAMMADI LIBRARY*, EDITED BY JAMES M. ROBINSON

To know thyself one has to first become conscious of all that one is. Luckily the ancient Egyptians had a system that allowed them to break down the vast spectrum of their inner worlds into ten bodies of light and ten layers, or veils, of existence. This system also ties in with the ten spheres found within the Tree of Life in the later Hebrew tradition.

Egypt is the heart and soul of the origins of Western culture and civilization. Much of the mathematics, alchemy, astronomy, astrology,

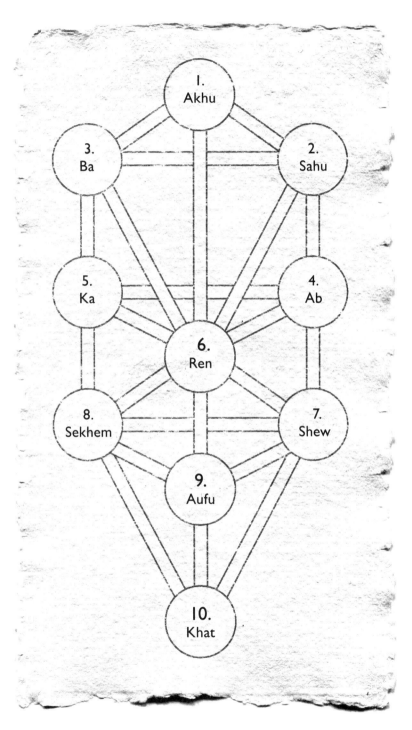

Tree of Life, the Ten Bodies of Light

and philosophy that were revered in ancient Greece came from Egypt, and even the American dollar bill has the Egyptian eye and pyramid emblazoned proudly on it. In a more spiritual vein Christ and many of his disciples were taught and initiated in Egypt, and they blended these teachings to create gnostic Christianity and the basis of the Knights Templar. Much of the Goddess culture was last established on a large scale in Egypt as well, before the downfall of the matriarchy there. One could say that the Egyptians have connected into, shared common wisdom with, and impacted our culture on almost every level.

The basis of the Egyptian art and science of the soul is a knowledge of the ten subtle bodies of light. To the Egyptians, just as we have our physical body, so too do we have nine other bodies that are absolutely real in other dimensions or wave bands of vibration. These additional nonphysical bodies enabled the Egyptians to sense, feel, navigate, and create many astounding feats of technology, science, and spirituality that still baffle us today.

These ten bodies are interpenetrating subtle bodies—layers of light, thought, feeling, color, and vibration emanating from the physical body into our planet, our solar system, and into the galaxy. These emanations were connected to the original source where the Egyptians felt their home was: Sirius, Orion, and the galactic center. When we look at the Tree of Life it is clear that the soul's path from divine desire to a fully embodied manifestation on Earth, journeys through ten spheres, each sphere creating yet another robe of light as the soul incarnates into ever denser dimensions.

The ten bodies effectively create and operate a holographic reality. With our intent we can bring all aspects of our energetic anatomy into a fully developed, coordinated, integrated, and unified being.

We can thus know ourselves by experiencing and becoming the ten in physical form. This path of initiation leads us into every facet of human and divine experience in order to become the fullness of our totality.

1. THE BODY OF MATTER: KHAT

The *khat* is our physical form, the empty vessel waiting to be filled with the animating forces of the other bodies of light. It is the door of the temple that opens into the experience of the other nine bodies, the key that unlocks the awareness of our multidimensionality. The khat is the container, which decays after death—the mortal, temporary part of us that was preserved in mummification by the ancient Egyptians. Interestingly enough we are told in the Egyptian Book of the Dead that during the process of death the khat becomes twenty-one grams lighter by the departure of the other bodies of light into formless realms.

Khat also means "form" or "appearance" and is the aspect of us that lives under the laws of time and space. It is the material temple where transformational change occurs, because it anchors and grounds the essence of our being onto Earth. This is essential to recognize as without khat we would not come to experience the totality of our human existence. Khat is the alchemical crucible that houses and holds together the transformation of all the other light bodies.

The Egyptians noted that as we journey through life and death on a spiritual path in our physical bodies, significant changes happen within the actual function of the physical body as it absorbs more light and transfigures itself into a vehicle of light. As it transfigures it raises its vibration and its ability to hold more light. This is also strengthened through the interface of the ka body, our holographic twin.

2. THE BODY OF LIFE: AUFU

We can come to know *aufu* as the totality of all the bodily systems and secretions, while the khat is the form, shape, and container. I see aufu as the "juicy intelligence" of the bodily liquids such as blood, lymph, water, sexual fluids, and all the mineral and metals within the body. The Egyptians believed that the lightness and clarity of the body's systems were a mark of spiritual growth, with the flesh being an indicator of how much light a person had brought into his or her physical body. The Egyptians did not denigrate or mutilate the body but rather worked with it so it could fulfill its purpose of transfiguration and light absorption.

To feed aufu properly is to eat foods that are life nourishing and green—such as raw, organic living foods and juices—drink good water, exercise, and breathe.

It is interesting to observe the connection of the *shew* (shadow) to the aufu, which can be seen in the dieting fads of today's world.

One of aufu's gifts is to provide us with the pleasures of this world through the senses. If the body is not well maintained and looked after then our appreciation of this world will diminish, and we will be less able to appreciate the beauty in nature and ourselves.

If aufu is looked after the heart is lighter, and we can make more peaceful, balanced, and heart-centered decisions. Aufu also affects the mind and emotions, because by nurturing aufu we love ourselves more, and this is when aufu sends out signals of contentment and peace to the other bodies, weaving them together in biological harmony.

Ways to Care for Khat and Aufu

1. Choose foods that are mostly raw, organic, fresh, and clean.
2. Choose supplements that nourish and enhance the body-mind-spirit connection.
3. Drink clean water, preferably alkalized, which helps the physical body to become more alkaline and thus allows more light into our cells.
4. Drink fresh and delicious juices and superfood smoothies.
5. Receive deep tissue massage (on the thirteen joints), and practice forms of yoga and exercise to help maintain the spiritual connection and alignment of muscle to spirit and light.
6. Sauna and get hydrotherapy regularly.

7. Exercise regularly (gym, tennis, cycling, walks).

8. Brush the skin to encourage lymphatic drainage.

9. Get nourishing sleep and rest.

10. Practice the awareness and experience of the five elements—earth, air, fire, water, and ether—and spend regular time in nature.

3. BODY OF FIRE: SEKHEM

Sekhem flows throughout all our subtle bodies and channels, chakras, meridians, and nadis as the creative force of the universe in motion. Sekhem, similar to shakti, is the creative power and flow of life force energy that connects body, mind, and soul. This is the living power of the Goddess, the creative force that manifests and creates. It is a passion and *desire* for life, and it takes life by the horns and rides with it. Sekhem can be sensual, sexual, rich, overflowing, and blissfully loving as well as powerfully transforming and at times ruthless in its destruction.

Sekhem is the creator and destroyer; she manifests in order to play, and her dance is one of delight. When we are in delight, free flowing, following our heart's desires and living them, then we are dancing in our full power and joy, and we are in her flow. Accomplishing your soul's purpose comes through the powerful prayer of sekhem merging with your heart-soul, the ab ba.

The main barriers to fully expressing the energy of sekhem are wounds found within the womb and hara. These wounds can be caused by sexual abuse and subsequent loss of connection to that area as well as the strictures of our culture and upbringing and early expectations or limits put on our behavior. Cultural straitjacketing of free expression and huge distortions and manipulations around sexuality and love have attempted to dampen our sekhem. Additionally, pressure to conform to what is considered right and acceptable in polite society, or in politically and spiritually correct circles, is what also keeps your sekhem under wraps or in a safe place. To express sekhem is to freely be who you are and to express your highest potential without fear of others' ridicule or limiting thoughts. Sekhem is the fuel for those who follow their hearts first and foremost, who live by her fiery fluidity and hunger for the fullness of life.

Ways to Care for Sekhem

1. Dance, act, and perform.
2. Practice pranayama and yoga.
3. Engage in extreme sports and adventure.
4. Engage in passionate and sensual lovemaking.
5. Travel and expand your experiences.
6. Go beyond your own limitations.
7. Follow your creative passions.
8. Have wild celebrations.
9. Work with archetypes.
10. Play, laugh, and have loads of fun!

4. BODY OF SHADOW: SHEW

The shew is our shadow body, which holds the painful memories, wounds, and injuries that we have hidden away from the light of our consciousness. By ignoring these elements and avoiding the processing of our own suffering the shadow further contracts into density. It wrings out whatever light there once was to a dry, barren, and bitter fury. Whenever someone touches the shew it bursts into life as a hellish rage and often leaves us saying, "I have no idea what came over me."

The shew works in the personal and collective unconscious, manifesting in our lives and relationships to show us what we have not healed, what we have not embraced, what needs our attention, what we are cut off from, and what we have ignored or rejected. However, the Egyptians understood that the shew, or shadow, also contains the potential to become our ally, teaching us lessons through adversity and clearly showing us what we have avoided, judged, and misperceived

In order to work with the shew effectively we need to gently guide it into a safe and nonjudgmental place, without the intention to rationalize or spiritualize the experience in any way. This is a temptation as the light and glory of the other bodies can blind us to our shadow. The human tendency is to identify most with light and power and not pay attention to the shadow, which lurks in the background. Yet the shadow is the source of our power.

It takes humility, honesty, and vulnerability to work authentically with the shew. By becoming humble and open to its suffering we can step-by-step begin to restore it to its original innocence.

Ways to Care for Shew

1. Communicate consciously.
2. Be transparent.
3. Practice humility.
4. Be nonjudgmental.
5. Engage in drama and acting.
6. Engage in physical activities to transmute the shew, such as martial arts and endurance training.
7. Create a safe space to communicate with the shew inwardly.
8. Retrieve the shew through journeywork and timeline healings.
9. Retrieve and heal childhood traumas and wounds.
10. Retrieve and heal relationship traumas and wounds.

5. BODY OF SOUND: REN

We first experience *ren* through the sound, tone, and expression of our own name and its resonance to us. Our name defines our relationship to the world and is the body of sound that defines our identity and form. When we name something we bring it into being. Our ren is our true spiritual name, the name that we resonate to most: the name of our soul. One of its purposes is to remind you of your essence when you forget. Ren carries within its vibration the sound of your soul, your God-given name, which creates resonance each time it is said and which holds great power once you learn what it is and how to use it.

Spiritual teachers throughout time have given their students names, yet today it is most important for you to remember your own name through prayer and meditation. When you are in a sacred site, temple, or in ceremony your original name can arise more quickly, because your soul is supported to open and delve deep into its essential sound vibration. When you sing spontaneously in abandon, letting go of yourself, then this sound—your soul song—can arise and unite you with all of creation.

There is the sense of rebirth when you rename yourself with the vibration and frequency coming from deep within you. In many ways this renaming ceremony can facilitate a born-again experience. To truly ground the experience I would advise you to make the change across the board—legally, emotionally, and practically. You can experiment with ren by sounding, writing, and imagining your current birth name and that of your soul and the idealized vibration that you wish to embody. Can you feel the differences inside when you sound these names? That is ren.

Ways to Care for Ren

1. Discover your true name.
2. Learn to write it in a way that portrays its essence.
3. Begin to anchor its vibration—by making changes legally, practically, and emotionally so it becomes real rather than fantasy.
4. Begin to use it with your friends and family.
5. Begin to use it in the technosphere (online and through the digital systems).
6. Record your voice repeating your name and listen when deeply relaxed.

7. Meditate upon your ren.

8. Journey through your ren and feel the frequencies that it contains.

6. BODY OF SPIRIT: KA

Our ka is the interface between the physical and all the other light bodies. It provides the container for our ability to travel and witness life when the physical body is not able to. The ka can provide distant healings, interactions, lucid dreams, and visions of other realities. Ka also provides an infrastructure for the body, emotions, and mind to actually exist. If you were to remove the ka, all subtle bodies would dissolve.

Ka is a matrix both within the body and outside the body. It can look like a clear quartz replica of the physical body, although the colors and hues may differ from person to person. Most of our feelings and thoughts are stored within the ka; it holds information and memory regarding our personal and collective existence.

When ka is well nourished we feel powerful, present, charismatic, alive, and delighted. We feel that we are able to achieve whatever we desire. Our motivation and clarity are high, and we have the power to move forward. We are actively engaged in the physical, and we enjoy life.

The ability to catalyze, create, and manifest more radiance and power emanates from the ka as well as the ability to desire and merge with another in conscious sexual practice. Ka is the imprint of that part of you that has a connection with the place that your physical body lives, with the objects you possess, and with the cords of connection and relationship you have with others. In the psychic realms ka imbues its imprint on its relationships and on objects it possesses. Each object and relationship we have holds an imprint of our ka, which stays with it, much as a fingerprint stays on a glass. Psychics have the capacity to pick up these residual traces of ka energy by touching the object.

Our ancestors knew and understood this power of the ka and thus chose to own few objects and possessions so as not to fritter away precious ka energy by spreading it randomly. When they died these ka or power objects, as they are known to shamans, were gathered together by family and friends and placed in the tomb with the mummified body so that the ba (soul) and ka would be able to complete their journey in the afterlife with this extra power. It is also important to note that these ka power objects were used extensively in life to boost the ka energy of the user at certain times, such as during rituals, important meetings, meditation, and lovemaking.

Ways to Care for Ka

1. Practice pranayama and yoga.
2. Practice meditation.
3. Ritualize the ending of relationships—cut cords and and take back your essence.
4. Ritualize moving and any endings or completions in life.
5. Do not accumulate too many objects and possessions or clutter.
6. Create time and space alone to integrate and be with your own energy.
7. Spend time in nature and consciously connect to the elements.
8. Take salt baths and natural spring washes to clear etheric debris.
9. Practice energetic lovemaking.

7. BODY OF LOVE: AB

The ab is the part of us that loves, deeply feels, and longs for union and intimacy. The voice of the ab forgives, inspires, frees, liberates, and imbues a transmission of love that can be felt and tasted. Here is where we experience the flow of love, the ability to trust, to discern, and to forgive.

The ab is the divine human heart—the foundational seat of the soul. It is the seat of your moral, ethical, and human values. It is the pure heart—the highest human expression of love. Ab manifests in every human heart as the impulse to connect deeply, to gently remove the veils of protection and distrust. Within the ab is the desire for intimacy, transparency, and real nakedness as the ab contains our untouched and untainted original innocence and purity of being. Here is where we discover humility, empathy, compassion, mercy, forgiveness, and charity.

Within the ab we discover our heart's voice and conscience. This part of us contains the capacity and willingness to vulnerably connect with our shadow in moments of radical honesty and conscious communication. This openness becomes the doorway to the soul (ba) and when we enter we are greeted by the power of love in its majestic fullness.

Love forever beckons us to become softer, sometimes through an accident, illness, loss, or a fright. In life we are all faced with incidents that teach us how to become less selfish and judgmental, more compassionate and generous. Some of us learn the lesson and manage to become milder, while others end up becoming even harsher than before. The only way to get closer to truth is to expand the heart so that it will encompass all humanity and still have room for more love.

Ways to Care for Ab

1. Write and read poetry.
2. Enjoy music and dance.
3. Engage in free expression.
4. Be honest and vulnerable.
5. Practice humility toward your feelings and the feelings of others.
6. Be transparent.
7. Be nonjudgmental.
8. Practice forgiveness.
9. Give yourself permission to feel.
10. Contribute proactively to the community—dharma/service.

8. BODY OF SOUL: BA

The ba is our soul, which over time can become anchored in our heart center, the ab. When the human heart ab and the soul ba merge they create a foundation to integrate, sustain, and activate the soul purpose and drive. Within our ba we find our soulful passions, desires, intentions, and dreams. This is the realm of our visions, our highest potential and drives. The emotions of longing, yearning, devotion, and rapture are discovered here in the ba. When we fully connect with the ba it becomes embodied and acted upon in the heart center of the ab.

Through the ba the most powerful experiences of God can be felt. When connected with the ba, prayer becomes an intimate expression and way of receiving divine love into our soul. The ba is the aspect of us that can receive God's love and gently filter it through the other bodies. By the pure nakedness found within the ba we can offer the most sincere and devotional prayers to our creator. The ba always remembers how to commune with God; it is the part of us that did not forget when we experienced the fall and separation.

Ba is your own unique, individual soul spark from the eternal flame of the universal soul. It is your first real introduction to unlimited, infinite, and unconditional love with no agendas, barriers, rules, dogmas, or restraints. Ba is the soul spark in each human being.

Ba is the spiritual manifestation and embodiment of your soul and its purpose. It holds the blueprint of your life and unique path. When you are in touch with your ba and its purpose many of the reasons for organized religion crumble, as you now know what you need and what to do. You have your own guidance and know your own rules and guidelines. You know yourself.

One of the most humbling experiences in life is when we remember what we came here to do and be, and why we decided to incarnate into the particular body, environment, parents, and country we chose in this lifetime. With this knowledge you can guide your life in the direction your ba longs for. You will be able to fulfill the deepest desires of your heart and soul and achieve your highest potential as a human being.

Finding your soul purpose is perhaps one of the most important tasks facing you today. Upon finding it and then consciously activating it, the whole world will conspire to help you achieve it, to lead you into the greatest love you can ever know.

Ways to Care for Ba

1. Practice prayer.
2. Pray to feel your connection with God.
3. Pray to feel all your feelings.
4. Bring God into your life (sacred union).
5. Love fully.
6. Always tell the truth.
7. Ask to know God's truth and laws.
8. Live by your soul, make all choices and decisions in accordance with your soul.
9. Practice soul retrieval.

9. BODY OF RESURRECTION: SAHU

In Egyptian *sa* means "life force," and *hu* is the flow of the universal sound similar to the sound *om*. Together this flowing of the life force within all beings, connected to the sound that underlies all life, reveals *sahu* within our physical structures. Simply put, sahu is the life force of the Source. You could say the God force.

As we enter sahu our blood, bones, spines, DNA, brain chakras, and physical structures all change as we become more crystalline, for sahu is the transfigured self. The body transfigures in order to contain the higher frequencies of light, and we will actually become a different type of human being, genetically, structurally, and consciously. The best-known recent example of this full transfiguration of the physical body into sahu was Jesus Christ after the Resurrection.

We access sahu when we become a God-conscious being living in human form, when we have evolved to a point where we are in the world but not of it, connected to Earth and its pleasures and joys while being connected to the Source of all that is. It is living heaven on Earth, being human and divine, embodying light into matter.

Sahu is the last evidence of physical form and the first evidence of eternity. It is where the temporary human form merges with the infinite. It is a luminous sheath of light that holds all our deepest codings within it, all the seals of all our previous initiations that help us to tap in to universal wisdom.

Sahu is the resurrection body; when fully developed it aligns with sekhem, the power of life. In order to access these both, the optimum route prescribed in Egypt was conscious lovemaking between a couple matched in love, as this involves the mixing of both human and divine energies and all the bodies of light.

Sahu is the marriage of earthly fertility, abundance, exuberance, and passion for life, with the mastery of stillness, silence, celestial wisdom, and power: the union of masculine and feminine as one flow of energy. When these two meet as one sahu is entered, and we live heaven on Earth, here in the body, we embody the richness of life brought into cosmic wisdom and light.

Ways to Care for Sahu

1. Practice stillness.
2. Consciously access the void, or emptiness.
3. Practice vipasana meditation.
4. Practice conscious lovemaking.
5. Meditate within the womb space.
6. Be in silence and blackness (resting in the dark equals black light).

7. Enter theta states.

8. Use flotation tanks or other methods of deep relaxation.

9. Use fasts, deep cleanses, and supplements to bring more light into the cells.

10. BODY OF GOD: AKHU

Akhu is the immortal Godself that manifests through the sahu, or immortal body. Beyond the ba and that which the *ba* dissolves and surrenders into, is akhu, the source of sahu. It is one's highest spiritual self, the immortal and imperishable spirit, uniting one's human self with one's highest self and with God.

In akhu one can take all the other bodies of light and consciously dissolve them back into their source when one is ready to realign and rebalance all bodies. The energies of akhu serve as a resurrection process and allow us to die into the deathless state, extinguishing all identification and being reborn into the next octave.

Akhu is the imperishable, immortal spirit.

Within akhu we find the great flame, which was known as the Holy Spirit to the apostles of Christ, who were anointed by akhu after the Resurrection with this flame blazing above their heads. The Egyptians saw akhu as the phoenix, the great blazing cosmic fire of resurrection, regeneration, and new creation.

The word *akh* comes from a root that means "to be effective, to have power and ability." Akh means that one has the ability to travel through and act in all the realms of this world as well as all others.

Akhu is the soul, or ba, surrendered back into God—the shining transfigured soul that is free to become anything at any time. This total fluidity means that one has total mastery and emptiness, which in turn allows one to access any frequency, any note on the scale of creation while simultaneously being unborn: not of the creation.

Akhu is a step beyond the ba soul, which is what most humans are striving for. Beyond the ba one has to surrender their soul to akhu, which means the absorption of the ba soul back into its source, that which has never been created and never been destroyed. Once the ba has returned to its source, then akhu flies free, able to perform anything required in the flow of creation at any moment through your vehicle.

Surrender is how akhu manifests.

Ways to Care for Akhu

1. Surrender.
2. Pray deeply to know and feel God.
3. Spend time alone in prayerful solitude.

ACCESSING THE TEN BODIES

 Sacred Initiation

■ Part One

Over a ten-day period come to know yourself through each of the ten light bodies. Tune in to one body at a time through the sacred arts of prayer, meditation, visualization, shamanic journeywork, and journal writing. Day by day bring your awareness to each aspect of yourself.

Throughout the day track your particular body, sense its whereabouts and what strengthens its essence. Commune with it directly—ask what it requires of you to integrate and strengthen it.

Give form to this robe of light that creates the vaster expression and awareness of your self. Write down all the knowledge and insight that you glean through this particular lens of your extended self.

■ Part Two

Over another ten-day period, if you are with your beloved meditate together holding your awareness within the same body of light. For example, one day you would both meditate on your own connection to your ab while simultaneously being aware of your beloved. This will begin the process of consciously bringing all ten of your bodies together.

Continue this practice every day until your have sat and communed together in all your bodies. Make sure you are in the same bodies at the same time. Continue for another ten-day period.

I move forward with trust and consciousness.

9

HEALING THE
THREEFOLD FLAME

I said to my soul, be still, and let the darkness come upon
  you
Which shall be the darkness of God.
I said to my soul, be still, and wait without hope
For hope would be hope for the wrong thing; wait without
  love,
For love would be love for the wrong thing; there is yet faith
But the faith and the love and the hope are all in the
  waiting.
Wait without thought, for you are not ready for thought:
So the darkness shall be the light, and the stillness the
  dancing.

T. S. ELIOT, "EAST COKER"

Now we enter the psychic realm that contains the ancient battle scars between the masculine and feminine principles. Even to this day these unconscious wounds get played out in modern relationships. These three wounds are located in at least one and possibly more of our ten bodies. Since receiving the wisdom contained in these three ancient stories I have been able to wrap words and understanding around these once elusive memories. I am confident that you will feel and receive the transmission held within these stories, and I know this will bring some relief and understanding as to why the genders have not trusted one another. Most important, through this deep understanding we can discover the ways and means to heal these age-old wounds that were seeded in ancient civilizations.

ANCIENT WOUNDS

My feeling is that until these great wounds from our historical past are authentically transformed, it does not matter how much work we put into our modern-day counseling and therapy sessions. Until the three ancient wounds are addressed they will still have the potential to haunt us. Our work is to heal the entire time line from original cause to present moment. With these stories we have the keys to access the age-old memories and transform the cause at its root—forever.

The Story of Separation in Lemuria (Love/Heart)

Once upon a time there was an ancient land called Lemuria, a place of innocence, tranquillity, and peace. A subtle realm of delicate beauty where freshly birthed souls still cooling from the fires of creation would tenderly undulate with the ecstasy of God's love.

These souls were androgynous and without form, simply existing as swaths of luminescent light that radiated throughout the whole cosmos as waves of divine love. Created from divine desire, the purity of their essence caused even the angelic kingdoms to prostrate in wonder at the sheer magnitude of God's work.

This subtle realm was connected to Earth, but not on Earth. It existed in another space, just a few octaves beyond the third dimension. Lemuria truly was a dominion of light and beauty, a place of pure paradise.

Eons passed, and deep within the nucleus of the soul a delicate shift began to take place. At a subtle level, unnoticeable at first, small signs of change began to take shape. Gentle little movements that contained the desire and impetus to separate began to occasionally quiver through the pure soul. From within the essence of the soul the finest mechanics began to orchestrate a process that would eventually separate the soul into two halves. This subtle movement was the original birth of duality—the tender division into masculine and feminine polarities.

The initial desire to separate was generated from within the essence that became born as masculine energy. There was a natural desire for it to know itself, to venture forward, to pioneer, to explore, and to experience what was beyond its current reality.

The essence that did not desire separation was the feminine principle. This part was totally fulfilled and content with its existence, and it did not understand or even feel this desire to go beyond what was already known.

As time passed the separation process continued, and a clearly defined masculine aspect began to seek total separation from the feminine. He could feel her resistance and reluctance to move forward into unknown territory, and this feeling triggered within him an even stronger urge to move on. By now a separate egoic identity was beginning to form, and its voice suggested to the masculine that he may have to go alone, without her. The ego whispered that she might attempt to hold him back from knowing himself and his place in the universe. For the first time, upon hearing these words, the masculine experienced fear that the feminine may indeed distract him from his divine destiny, and so in response to his fear he further contracted and placed his will in favor of a complete separation.

Within the feminine a huge energy of abandonment began to be born and be felt throughout her awareness. She did not understand the desire to move beyond and to know more, and for the first time she experienced fear *that her other half would leave her completely. In the deepest of places she despised his desire to move away from her, and therefore she withheld her loving emanations from him. The egoic nature of the feminine was also being born as a range of sensory feelings—from the terrifying fear of abandonment to an endless icy despair. The feminine immediately contracted at such feelings, and together at the same time the masculine and feminine witnessed the beginnings of a physical tear within their soul.*

In unison they screamed at the appearance of the first tear, and a wave of terror moved through them both. They knew they were moving in to unknown territory, and suddenly they weren't sure whether they could survive without one another. All of these realizations swam into their consciousness, causing an overwhelming sense of disorientation and fear. The experience of this excruciating pain caused them to instinctively move away as fast as they could from the rip in their existence. The severity of this impulsive action inevitably led to an even deeper rip. In near paralysis they looked at one another across the canyon that was already forming between them. This last gaze held a certain coldness, laced with a deep and seemingly irreparable sense of regret. Within this moment time and space stood still. With one last glimpse of one another they sided with their fear and simultaneously turned their backs on each other. They powerfully pushed against the boundaries of their essence to further forge the full separation of their soul into two distinct halves. This separation was the birth of the original masculine and feminine principles on Earth. In that moment there was a twofold manifestation. Not only did they find themselves separated into two distinct selves, but the diminishing of their soul light caused yet another occurrence—the creation of a body of flesh. Now not only were they separated by space but also by form.

—————— ♦ ——————

For the healing and transformation of this soul wound it is important to enter into the story and feel how it touches you and unfolds inside you. This wound lives within the boundaries of the heart in both men and women. It is the guardian that stands before you suggesting the need and desire to protect yourself from love. As you move toward full heartfelt union this will be the main wound that resurfaces. There will be myriad reasons why it's wise to protect yourself, to not give everything to love.

The truth is what you withhold from love is exactly what you withhold from yourself. We imagine that a broken heart is a heart that has become wounded from love, when in actual fact it is a heart that is being held hostage from loving fully.

These wounds of abandonment and the fear of being held back and controlled are still painfully alive today. With this story of the original cause we are given the keys to heal this injury at its root. In this way waves of healing will have the ability to travel both forward into the present day and back into the past.

Remember to feel both the masculine and feminine wounds inside you so you can intuit the story from each perspective. Human beings have evolved to such a degree now that both the masculine and feminine principles live within us. However, at the beginning of time this was not the case, nor was it the intended desire.

The Story of the Abuse of Power in Atlantis (Wisdom/Consciousness)

Once upon a time there was an ancient land called Atlantis, a place of elegance, evolution, and creative abundance where a group of highly advanced souls were beginning to radically explore the boundaries of human understanding. Atlantis was fast becoming a place renowned for its evolved and highly sophisticated freethinkers who were on the cutting edge of discovery and experimental breakthrough.

It was a time in Earth's history when the energies were naturally moving into a more masculine polarity. However, the civilization in Atlantis marked the first time that humankind had experienced one of these earthly cycles. Little did they know that the shift from one polarity to the other was a natural and harmonious wave of energy. This wave contained the opportunity to know and embody the divine masculine principles: to know the truth of God and the laws of his universe.

Within Atlantis men and women who leaned more toward the masculine principle were entering a phase of development that was truly uncharted. There seemed to be a tremendous evolutionary spirit soaring through the fields of science, math, and both the universal and biological laws of creation.

The groups involved in these pursuits were consumed with a spiritual fire that began to sustain them from the inside. There was almost no need to sleep, eat, or do anything else, as their passion for radical thinking and experimentation was all that they lived for. It was as if they had tapped in to a new power that the rest of Atlantis had yet to discover.

As time passed this hunger for more and more wild experimentation took root and grew. However, outside these circles there was a growing concern that the experiments and explorations were unbalanced and that there was no responsible authority guiding or overseeing the work. From within the main scientific groups radical offshoots were springing up in an attempt to take the experimentation to the next quantum level. Often without permission these groups would simply take it upon themselves to fund and oversee their work by trial and error until their visions succeeded in reality. Doubts and fears were beginning to rise from within the greater communities of Atlantis. People gathered behind closed doors as they whispered their concerns and feelings of unease. The people wanted to know what exactly was going on within the walls of these laboratories where no one seemed to be overseeing the progress of these now highly secretive and powerful groups of scientists.

The feminine principle in Atlantis, representing the people who worked with the land and found their spirituality within the elements of nature, began to look upon the masculine principle with a sense of dread and foreboding. She noticed how these people were abandoning their love for Earth and discarding their nature-based spirituality for what they were calling a new form of spirituality—science. These scientists were declaring that they were listening to the voice of God and that they had become his special spokespeople. They declared that the old spiritual way where everyone was equal and able to speak and listen to God no longer existed.

"God can no longer be found within nature. God can now only be found within science. It is God that is leading this experimentation. He has appointed us as his priests to speak and act on his behalf," was the voice of the masculine.

These radical freethinkers were introducing a new form of spirituality, and for the first time in human history the idea of a spiritual hierarchy was born on Earth. This new religion stated that God could no longer be accessed through the old ways and that if you wanted to connect with him you would have to go through a priest of Atlantis.

This was shocking and unnerving news to the rest of Atlantis. It brought about a great deal of unrest and an immediate divide between the masculine and feminine principles. This increased the growing distrust and rampant fear, because the very essence of the feminine principle was being questioned at a fundamental level. Those who carried the feminine principle within their hearts were being challenged to prove the need or place for the existence of the feminine in this brave new world that was being born.

It was a frightening time. Dark clouds were beginning to gather as the masculine principle began to depart from its original balance and reach distorted and destructive levels of power. Refusing to listen to the growing concerns of the people, the masculine turned his back and returned to his work, where he now admitted that in many ways he was playing God.

Rumors spread like wildfire through the streets and homes of Atlantis. There were stories of how mutant babies were being born who were half human and half animal, and how they were attempting to bend the laws of nature to produce a fifth element. There was also talk of a brand-new power being created that was being produced as a result of creating mini black holes and then exploding them.

This news created a deep-seated fear within the feminine as she knew these types of experimentation should not be happening. These scientific experiments were acutely dangerous and had the power to destroy the whole of Atlantis and possibly the entire Earth. And yet when it came to voicing her opinion, the feminine found that the scientific evidence and clever calculating responses from the masculine undermined and humiliated her concerns.

"You know nothing about this, woman, and it does not concern you. You are no longer needed. We have grown beyond your understandings, and your power is obsolete. Go back to your house and refrain from attempting to question our authority. You have no voice here."

She was not only ignored but ridiculed as well. This open mockery left her feeling powerless and without expression. She attempted again and again to look for ways into the heart of the masculine with the hope that he would see sense and stop his misuse of power. The more she came forward the stronger and more arrogant he became. Over time she became silenced and in many ways seen as infertile, menopausal, and not needed anymore. The majority of people in Atlantis foolishly believed all that was being told to them and gave their power away to the priests of this new scientific god. Only a handful of people stayed true to the feminine and kept her ways alive.

This handful of people powerlessly looked on, totally unable to speak of their concerns, because no one was willing to listen to them. The people of Atlantis had become blind to the power that was manipulating them, imagining it to be the voice of this glorious new evolutionary spirit that promised the Earth in more ways than one. The feminine principle could see the distortion and the corruption, but she was unable to do anything about it, while the masculine basked in his own egoic glory.

The feminine principle sank to an all-time low, while the masculine spirit soared to dizzying and macabre new heights. Atlantis was fast becoming a circus, a spectacle of twisted and wretched abuses of power and manipulation. This once glorious land had become a hotbed of corruption and arrogance. A land of self-appointed demigods who had developed a blood lust for their own glory.

——————————— ◆ ———————————

For the healing and transformation of this soul wound it is important to enter into the story and feel how it touches you and unfolds inside you. This wound lives within the boundaries of the mind—the consciousness—in both men and women. It is the guardian that stands before you suggesting the need and desire to protect yourself from the abuse of power from the masculine principle. It is important to remember that men can feel this wound if their women have a strong masculine side. As you move toward full conscious union this will be the main wound that resurfaces. There will be myriad reasons that come up as to why it's wise to protect yourself, to not share your inner world, to not give the whole truth. Be aware that the flavor of this wound orbits around distrust, suspicion, and the inability to speak out or confront obvious corruption and distortion. There is a feeling that only you can see the truth and that everyone else is either blind or in denial. Fear of authority and/or a strong aggressive masculine energy are the ramifications of this wound.

These wounds from the abuse of power and feminine disempowerment are still painfully alive today. With this story of the original cause we are being given the keys to heal this injury at its creation so that the waves of healing have the ability to travel both forward into the present day and back into the past, thus healing the root cause.

The Story of the Deceit
and Denial in Ancient Egypt
(Power/Sexuality)

Once upon a time in the earliest days of ancient Egypt a new era was being birthed based upon the principles of beauty, sensuality, and a passionate celebration of the sacred and magical arts. Egypt was fast becoming a place where highly advanced souls were exploring the world of magic, alchemy, and spiritual awareness. It was a time of wondrous discovery and the introduction of new ideas regarding astronomy, cosmology, and how to marry sexuality with spirituality.

This was a time in Earth's history when the energies were naturally moving into a more feminine polarity. However, this was the first time humankind had experienced one of these earthly cycles move into the feminine principle. Little did they know that the shift from one polarity to the other was a natural and harmonious wave of energy that contained the opportunity to know and embody the Divine Feminine principles—to know the truth of the Goddess and the laws of her universe.

Within Egypt men and women who leaned more toward the feminine principle were entering a phase of development that was truly unchartered. There seemed to be a tremendous evolutionary spirit soaring through the realms of mystery and magic and the spiritual and sexual ways of expressing this energy within a celebration of the body. This was manifesting as new forms of dance, performance, bodily decoration, and dress as well as the creation of various magical objects, potions, ointments, and oils.

The groups consumed with these desires seemed to be almost possessed by a spiritual fire that sustained them from the inside. There was no need to sleep, eat, or do anything else as their passionate appetite for magical experiences and the ability to be able to harness the powers of the universe reached an all-time high. It was as if these people had tapped in to a new power that the rest of Egypt had yet to discover.

As time passed these people went on to become the priests and priestesses of ancient Egypt, assuming a spiritual role and becoming a mouthpiece for the whole country. The priests used the Great Pyramid on the Giza Plateau as their spiritual headquarters, while the priestesses took the domain of the Isis Pyramid as their temple space. Because this was a time in history where the feminine principle was becoming more dominant, there was an inclination to share and reveal the processes of this spiritual abundance so that its prosperity could flood the land. Soon the whole of ancient Egypt was working with the feminine spirit by using various forms of ritualistic magic and ceremony. Almost overnight Egypt became a legendary, exotic, and mystical land that thrived with incredible abundance and celebration.

As time passed this feminine spirit began to naturally become stronger and stronger. The priestesses wove through the crowds, drenched in finery, as they trailed wafts of erotic enticement behind them. In small pockets of the masculine community voices began to express some concerns that the priestesses were reaching dizzying heights with their magical abilities and that perhaps it was not wise for women to have so much power. In some respects this was true, for indeed these high priestesses seemed to be filled with an otherworldly glow as their pure sexual attraction became uncomfortably seductive to some.

Whenever anyone challenged the priestesses they were met with an intoxicating beauty and love that immediately undermined their argument. This heightened attraction—although incredibly enticing and mesmerizing—was beginning to be hated, loathed, and seen with the eyes of suspicion. The masculine was unable to hold or fully embody his energy when in the presence of a priestess, because he was immediately disarmed and rendered impotent.

Word got back to the priests of ancient Egypt that the masculine spirit of Egypt was growing impatient and that action needed to be taken.

Within the walls of the Great Pyramid voices spoke of the same unrest within the magical worlds and how it was now time to address these issues. They couldn't understand why they could not reach the same magnificent outcomes as the priestesses when they too were working with the same magical principles and laws of alchemy. Male competitive spirit had been born, and along with it waves of resentment were building. More time passed as the priests looked on with suspicious eyes and growing concerns. Secret meetings were happening inside the Great Pyramid, where the masculine gathered and discussed the various ways in which they could take down the power of the feminine.

One of the ways in which the priests and priestesses worked was a twice daily sacred ceremony that happened every sunrise and sunset. At these times a priest and priestess would come together in the third pyramid (that we can still see) in the Giza Plateau and perform sacred union. This was a form of sex magic that involved the invoking and embodying of the feminine and masculine oversouls of the enigmatic Isis and Osiris. Two pure beings of ancient Egypt, Isis and Osiris, had originally led Egypt to its glorious heights of magic and power and had now passed from the physical world to continue on their soul adventure in the spiritual world. This twice daily ceremony performed by a priest and priestess was originally a deeply sacred and glorious act of merging spirituality with sexuality. It was performed with the highest of intention as a way of radiating the energy of sacred union into the land and its people, enhancing fertility and harmony.

However, the disgruntled priests now had developed a plan through which they could distort and control the energies of sacred union and harness its potency for an altogether different agenda.

On one particular morning a priest walked across the Giza Plateau with the intention to take from the priestess the sacred and vital energy stored within her womb. As he entered the sacred union pyramid the priestess immediately sensed a grave distortion and change in energy from within her masculine counterpart and adjusted accordingly. All this happened within nanoseconds. What she had done was to swiftly move her energy from within her womb up into her third eye for safekeeping, leaving her womb empty, barren from her sumptuous bounty.

The priest also recognized that a powerful alteration in energy had occurred, but neither of them said anything. That morning, under instruction of the head priest, he had partaken of a similar movement of energy. He had moved all this energy from his third eye as a response to the growing convictions that the priestesses were attempting to control them in some way through their thoughtforms and consciousness. He had sunk all his essence down into his groin, into his sexuality, with the desire and intention to steal the feminine essence from within the womb of the priestess. They faced one another knowing deep inside that a hidden agenda was at play. Yet both of them denied that they contained a secret. Both of them denied knowledge of such deceit.

The priest found an empty womb despite the priestess appearing to be present and loving. She had purposely withheld and mystified the process by overcloaking her energies to appear normal and open. She held the intention of looking inside his consciousness to find out why this was happening. She wanted to see and read his suspicions. She wanted to read his mind.

When she peered inside him she discovered emptiness, because he had done the same act. He had moved his energy from his third eye into the groin. He too was hiding from her and appearing present and open. Checkmate. Their suspicion and fear of one another deepened as it now seemed that it was imperative to protect themselves from one another in the sexual act.

It was here, in this moment, that the energies of deceit and denial entered the sacred union ceremonial process, which foolishly leaked into the ritualistic prayer to emanate throughout the land and its entire people. Within days the collective consciousness had begun to receive the distorted energies of the polluted sacred act. Twice daily different priests and priestesses would meet after being given the instruction to move their energies and to withhold their vital essence from the ceremony. And twice daily this energy would be spread throughout the whole of Egypt. It was only a matter of time before the great downfall would occur and bring Egypt to its knees.

━━━━━━━ ◆ ━━━━━━━

For the healing and transformation of this soul wound it is important to enter into the story and feel how it touches you and unfolds inside you. This wound lives within the boundaries of your sexuality—power—in both men and women. It is the guardian that stands before you suggesting the need and desire to protect yourself from being used or controlled within the sexual act and to protect yourself from being in relationship. This is the wound and suspicious fear of the dark feminine. It is important to remember that women can feel this wound if their man has a strong feminine side. The fear is that he will abuse his sexual power and art of seduction. As you move toward full sexual union this will be the main wound that resurfaces. There will be myriad reasons why you believe it is wise to protect yourself, to not share your full sexuality, to not give the whole of yourself. Be aware that the flavor of this wound orbits around deceit, suspicion, and the ability to even deny its existence, when you both (or one of you) knows that it is happening. Fear of sexuality and its wild chaotic nature and/or fear of a strong feminine energy are the ramifications of this wound.

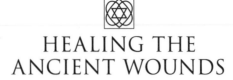

HEALING THE
ANCIENT WOUNDS

These wounds from denial and deceit and masculine disempowerment are still painfully alive today. People are still coming together to make love with this abnormal configuration of energy within their DNA. Women today are still stuck in their heads, and men are still stuck within their sexual center. We meet one another inside this emptiness with a deep psychic wound of fear that the other will steal our essence and life force. With the story of the original cause we are given the keys to heal this injury at its root and creation so that the waves of healing have the ability to travel both forward into the present day and back into the past.

Sacred Initiation

Begin to feel into these wounds first by yourself, writing down your contemplations and insights into how they show up in your present life. Again feel into both the masculine and feminine storylines.

Then begin to share them openly with your partner, making sure that both of you are openly discussing and revealing their patterning inside you.

Finally, choose three dates when it is a full moon (for dissolving) to perform a ceremony where you will release your participation in these wounds, either by yourself if you are single or together if in a relationship. It is important to allow yourself to grieve these wounds down to their causal level. This means to examine the hook into the wound that you still carry. There will be an emotional reason as to why you can still feel them as you read the story or listen to them on my *Wounds of Love* album.

You need to feel into your own personal hook and keep dropping down through the layers of your consciousness until you reach the fullness of your energetic connection with it. Remember to scan and be aware of all ten bodies. Your sacred initiation is to search throughout your entirety, retrieving all aspects of unknown and suppressed consciousness and emotionality surrounding these wounds.

Then finally, through an act of ceremony, release your own part in them.

Use your imagination, and remember you now have ten bodies to partake in your magical work.

I move forward with trust and consciousness.

DIVINE MARRIAGE
The Tenth Month

And yet neither Solomon nor Sheba became a consort of the other, for they were equals, each a sovereign being, with charge over his and her own domain and destiny.

KATHLEEN MCGOWAN,
"THE LEGEND OF SOLOMON AND SHEBA"

As we enter into the final stages of our journey it is here at the pinnacle of our adventure together where "you must increase and I must decrease" (John 3:30). Here at the threshold of the steps leading to the unspeakable sanctity of sacred union, or hieros gamos, I shall diminish into the mystery. I will lead you toward the temple doors, but I cannot enter. Over the past nine months you have been crafted, carved, and cultivated into the living emanation of the threefold flame. What was once a vision has emerged as a tangibly felt essence within your being. The last step is the one that leads you into the unknown, and it is something held between you, your beloved, and God.

All that I can do for you is to outline the process and bring to your attention the seven sacraments. My hope is to prepare you on every level—physically, sexually, emotionally, mentally, and soulfully.

CHOOSING THE RIGHT TIME AND SPACE
FOR THE BRIDAL CHAMBER

You will need a beautiful, healing, gentle, and womblike space where you will not be disturbed for a full lunar cycle. It would be wise to choose a space that has supportive and positive energy. I would choose an environment in nature with plenty of natural light and fresh air, close to water for bathing. Look for the presence of the five elements—earth, water, fire, air, and ether—or create them in microcosm for yourselves.

It is also important that this space be as clean as possible from electromagnetic frequencies: one that has the least amount of electrical smog from computers, TVs, mobile phones, and wireless gadgets. This is why I always suggest a natural environment as far away as possible from the urban world. When my beloved and I entered this process we both agreed to not bring our computers, phones, or any electrical devices into the sacred space. We made sure that we weaned ourselves off them *before* entering the full sacred union process; otherwise we would have brought addictive energy into the sacred environment, which could have interfered with the subtleties of the ritual.

The reason you are looking for an environment where you will not encounter any other people is because you are entering a soul reunification process. This is a highly intense energetic alchemy that involves the weaving together of the essence of two human beings in the known presence of God. Just for a moment imagine how refined and subtle this work is going to be. For days and nights you and your beloved have been together in the most exquisite flows of incredibly pure and high-frequency energy, when suddenly another human being comes into your environment. Can you feel the impact of that? It is important to be aware that when we reach the energetic embodiment of our original innocence even the thought of another can powerfully tilt or taint the field. This is why it is important to know (and own) thyself. Furthermore, with the growing awareness of our ten light bodies we meet one another in the fullness of our presence, knowing that whatever one does, the other shall feel it.

Now we need to look at the timings for such a significant and life-changing event to take place. The process is a monthlong initiation that begins on a new moon and ends on the eve of the next new moon. In truth a lunar cycle takes 29.5305882 days. However, let us agree to thirty days to complete our ritual. In the yogic schools we know that a woman responds instantaneously to the lunar rhythms felt within her body. Every two and a half days the moon's energy triggers another facet of her personality, giving the impression that she is changeable and unpredictable. Both partners are invited to surrender into the lunar rhythm as it is the feminine principle that will become paramount in both genders for this ritualistic process to work.

New moons are the most perfect times for new beginnings and, according to Kabbalists, the most opportune time for the creation and birth of a project. This is why we begin at the new moon. I would advise against beginning this work six weeks before either of your birth-days. This goes back to the fifty-two-day Saturn period just before your birthday, as explained in the first chapter.

As you move toward the full moon expect the energies to build and intensify as this is simply the nature of the full moon and her effect upon us. Any shadow or hidden elements that may arise could become more prevalent during this time. This is the gift of the full moon. My advice to you is to use this moon as a gateway to release any buildup of tension, blocks, or resistances to going deeper; or unconscious feelings and sensations that you cannot put your finger on. Give these shadowy aspects form, be it through the written word, sacred sound, or by your own vocal expression. Make a ritual on the full moon for these elements to be banished. Have a bonfire, if safe to do so, as you make offerings to the five elements. This will assist you with your process and the removal of all obstacles, seen and unseen.

> They stayed in the bridal chamber for the full cycle of the moon in the energies of trust and consciousness, allowing nothing to come between them in their union, and it is said that the secrets of the Universe were revealed through them.
>
> Together, they found the mysteries that God would share with the world, for those with the ears to hear.
>
> KATHLEEN McGOWAN, "THE LEGEND OF SOLOMON AND SHEBA"

BECOMING THE QUEEN AND KING

In the above quote we read how the sacred union between Solomon and Sheba was conceived and consummated by both a king and a queen. When researching this subject, everywhere I looked I discovered this terminology of monarchy or royal blood when referring to the beloveds who entered into this initiation. I do not believe this had anything to do with being a king or a queen in the external world, but rather it refers to a state of being that reflects the internal nobility of that person.

Even when we internally explore the archetypes of both king and queen we can feel the shift within us. This energetic shift is important, and it needs to become one that we embody as we step into the process. What does this really mean?

Sitting on Her Throne

When a woman takes to her throne as a majestic and noble queen there are qualities and insights that are revealed and sworn to.

1. She now becomes a servant in service to love, truth, and God.
2. To sit upon her throne could sometimes be pleasurable or

painful, yet to a queen neither is of her concern. Her throne is her domain and destiny, and it is her sovereign duty to govern her affairs and the administration of her love, power, and wisdom in all matters.

3. She can no longer bend for anyone or anything that is not serving her highest destiny; she sits powerfully in who she truly is and opens with love and humility to expand even beyond her own perceptions.

4. She is irresistible at every moment and extends the invitation to love by remaining in service of it. She is clear that she no longer goes looking for love or approval outside herself as she has claimed herself within. The queen knows that she is the source, the infinite fountain of this most precious elixir. She has cultivated her own inner marriage of masculine and feminine energies, and it is in celebration of her divine marriage with her soul half that she enters the sacred union process.

5. When she decides to invite a partner into her life she only chooses a king. This king recognizes his queen and bows to her in love, devotion, and the commitment to be of service to her highest destiny, his highest destiny, the highest destiny of the partnership, and the greatest of service to the larger community.

Sitting on His Throne

When a man takes to his throne as a majestic and noble king there are qualities and insights that are revealed and sworn to.

1. He now becomes a servant in service to truth, love, and God.

2. To sit upon his throne could sometimes be powerful or fearful, yet to a king neither is of his concern. His throne is his domain and destiny, and it is his sovereign duty to govern his affairs and the administration of his love, power, and wisdom in all matters.

3. He no longer suffers fools gladly and will not bend for anyone or anything that is not serving his highest destiny. He sits powerfully in who he truly is and opens to the love and humility to expand even beyond his own perceptions.

4. He is powerful at every moment and extends the invitation to be true by remaining in service of truth. He is clear that he no longer goes looking for truth outside himself as he has claimed it within. The king knows that he is the source, the infinite fountain of this most precious elixir. He has cultivated his own inner marriage of his masculine and feminine energies, and it is in celebration of his divine marriage with his soul half that he enters the sacred union process.

5. When he decides to invite a partner into his life he only chooses a queen. This queen recognizes her king and bows to him in love, devotion, and commitment to be of service to his highest destiny, her highest destiny, the highest destiny of the partnership, and the greatest of service to the larger community.

THE SACRED UNION, OR HIEROS GAMOS, RITUALISTIC CEREMONY

This ritual is based on an understanding of holographic principles and realties. Once you step into the space the hologram opens up, revealing a multilayered experiential dominion. This is precisely why we have taken the slow and methodical path, harnessing and anchoring our own understandings of multidimensional realties. Working diligently through our wounds and injuries of love as we transformed any potential obstructions early on, rather than during the process. Unhealed wounds would have obstructed the ritual, causing powerful explosions of emotional energy that would most likely have prevented the ceremony from being completed. As we progressed over the past nine months we have become aware of the seven gates of our sexuality, the five forms of love, and the ten light bodies of our consciousness. Add all these together and we have twenty-two (7 + 5 + 10 = 22).

Hold that figure for a moment.

Let's take another look at the kabbalistic Tree of Life. We are told that this mystical symbol is based on two pillars, like those that stood at the entrance to the Temple of Solomon. The Pillar of Mercy is on one side, and the Pillar of Severity is on the other. However, when I look at the Tree of Life, I see three pillars. Not only that, but when I look deeper still I see the entire hologram of sacred union. I sense that the Tree of Life is a map, route, and template that reveal the mechanics and mystery of the soul reunification process. I see the three pillars based on the threefold flame of power, love, and wisdom. I see the ten sephiroth as the ten light bodies ranging in vibrational frequency as sheaths of light. I also see the pentagram of the five wounds of love that guard the five forms of love (agape, eros, philia, storge, and rapture).

Finally I see *twenty-two* pathways that link the whole Tree of Life together. Twenty-two being a master number, is the number associated with Mary Magdalene. It is also the total number of initiations we have taken leading up to this point (7 + 5 + 10 = 22).

The Tree of Life depicts our entirety from the most refined subtle swathes of existence to the coarse realties of the physical body and its place on Earth. When we consciously bring together our Tree of Life with our soul half there is a powerful magnetic attraction, and the soul halves literally line up and prepare to fuse together. By merging the ten bodies and seven gates with the five forms of love a Jacob's ladder simultaneously appears, revealing once again the way into paradise, or nirvana. We fell from the heavenly garden because we wanted to know what the gods know. We chose to experience separation from God and from our soul half. On the horizon of our evolution, as the sun rises into this new era, the path of sacred reunion reveals our step-by-step process of reunification.

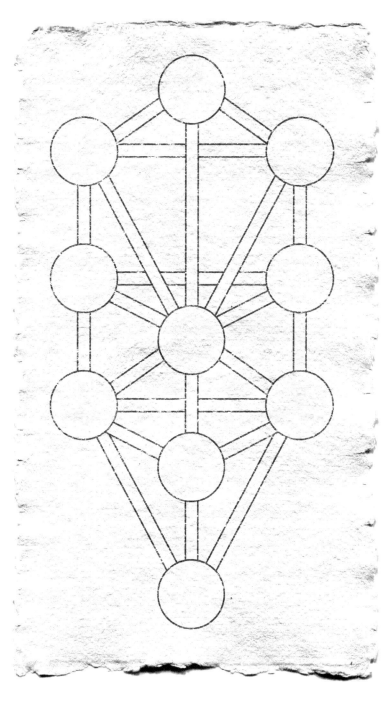

Tree of Life

The Feminine and Masculine Principles in Sacred Union

The feminine principle is brought into the process and embodied through lovemaking, massage, bodily movement, delicious high-vibrational feasts (raw, vegan, or vegetarian), deep relaxation, sensuality, intimacy, walking in nature, swimming, playfulness, creativity, joyful living, and the fluid ease of being. The role of the feminine is to keep the lovemaking consistent and lasting. This doesn't mean that you stay in bed for thirty days, although you can if you choose. What I mean is that you stay in the aroused state of emotional connectedness and intimacy. By constantly generating the lovemaking energies and channeling them through the five senses via touch, words, smell, taste, and vision you will begin to harness and build the alchemical energies. The most powerful, undeniable dimensional gateways are found within the flows of love. The deepest spectral ranges of experience will be found when both beloveds pass through the various "wormholes" that open up when you enter the theta states during and after lovemaking.

The masculine principle keeps a gentle form of structure within the shared consciousness of the beloveds. He is brought into the process and embodied through the awareness of the hologram, the coming together at the start of every day with the awareness of a slight shift in attention. The masculine navigates the dimensional spaces that both beloveds move through, highlighting and making note of the experiences that are occurring. The masculine is loosely witnessing the entire process while knowing the times when he is being asked to surrender, to release all that he thinks he has learned. The more he lets go, the more profound his territory.

The Threefold Flame in Sacred Union

For thirty days you will surrender into the most unknown mysteries of lovemaking, emotional connectedness, and soul braiding. During this entire lunar cycle you are being invited to lose yourself completely as you succumb to something far greater than your desire to reunify. Every day and night you will be fanning the flames of power, love, and wisdom through your various means of lovemaking, intimacy, and visioning

Take all that you have learned into the ceremony—the use of all seven gates, the engagement and activation of all five flows of love, and the faceted aspects of all ten bodies.

Finally and most important, bring to life the consistent awareness of and active participation with the masculine and feminine faces of God. For the next thirty days you are being asked to sleep with God, make love with God, eat with God, sing to God, pray to God, dance for God, massage with God, write to God, and more. In fact everything is done with God; there is no place where God is not actively being adored, loved, and included.

When looking at the few extant writings on hieros gamos we discover that the masculine and feminine aspects of God were always powerfully evoked before the ritual begins and also at the start of every lovemaking experience. With King Solomon and the Queen of Sheba we are told that they invoked the masculine and feminine presence of God, known in the Jewish tradition as El and Asherah. El was the fatherly consort and masculine principle, while Asherah was known as the Queen of Heaven and the feminine consort. In the Christian tradition it is suggested that Jesus Christ called upon the Logos to merge with him, while Mary Magdalene called forth the energies of Sophia. It is also well documented in the sexual practices of ancient Egypt that the energies of Isis and Osiris are invoked before all mystical rites of initiation.

This is something that needs to be discussed. Which tradition calls to you? I recommend that you sincerely pray with a pure heart to God to invoke the masculine and feminine qualities of God. I do not feel that invoking deities, entities, or spirits of smaller gods and goddesses would be a wise move as whatever you evoke shall become merged with you in the soul-braiding process. What is crucial in this process is that you are working with the law of three. For alchemy to take place there has to be three beings, three elements. In the case of sacred union the elements are man, woman, and God. The third being must be introduced for this work to be successful; it cannot be achieved without the presence of God.

Applying the Seven Sacraments

The seven sacraments are loosely based upon the Christian ideals of baptism, chrism, holy matrimony, Holy Communion, confession, ordination, and anointing of the sick. According to the Christian faith the seven sacraments are known as the seven mysteries that invoke the flow of grace to be freely received within humankind. These are the same sacraments that I have applied since I was a child, and I still facilitate them when holding a group or when in an intimate space. The very first time I performed them I *knew* that these outward actions held within them the presence of divine truth. There was no denying the tangibly felt presence of what we know of as the Holy Spirit moving through the sacramental motion into the awaiting and rapturous soul.

Baptism

Baptism represents death, interment, life, and resurrection. When we plunge our heads under the water, as in a sepulcher or pool of water, the old persona becomes completely drowned and buried. When one emerges from the water the new soul has been born into a reality cleansed of all error. Baptism is a ritual that is not only found in the Christian tradition but throughout the majority of all mystical, spiritual, and religious traditions. Among them we find the Druidic tradition, the mystery religions of Greece and Rome, the Hindu religion, and the ancient Egyptian Mystery Schools, where every temple had a sacred pool where the worshippers were baptized.

My recommendation would be to perform a baptism on the first day that you enter the sacred union process. Ideally you would have a river or pool of natural water near by. Otherwise a bath or shower will suffice. Your intentions need to be in alignment with the dissolving of all and any negative energies and self-sabotaging obstacles. Make sure that you submerge yourself completely and that the top of your head gets covered with water. This is a beautiful ceremony to perform for one another. Take your time; make a day of it. Make it sacred and holy.

Chrism

Chrism, or confirmation, is a type of second baptism with oil instead of water. Oil is the symbolic equivalent of fire as it is fire's fuel. Chrism actually corresponds to the baptism by fire of the Holy Spirit. The word *chrism* means "oil" or "anointing" in Greek. The ritual of anointing is used not only in confirmation but also in extreme unction and consecration of priests, priestesses, kings, queens, temples, statues, and so on.

Chrism corresponds to the fiery avatar of the Holy Spirit as a sort of *vajra,* or meteorite falling from the skies over the apostles during Pentecost. It imparts charisma—grace—and the gift of abundance and healing powers. In conclusion one might say that chrism or anointing corresponds to the baptism by fire of the Holy Spirit (feminine) whereas the baptism by water corresponds to the one of the father (masculine).

My recommendation is to perform a chrism on the first night that you enter the sacred union process as you invoke for the first time the masculine and feminine presence of God to enter into the process with you. This is a very big deal! This is truly one of the holiest ceremonies that you will ever do in your whole life. Please take your time as you bring your full awareness to the enormity of what you are about to enter into and work with. Please perform this ceremony with sincerity, purity, and humility. Ideally you need a selection of anointing oils such as spikenard (the oil that Mary Magdalene used to anoint Christ), frankincense, myrrh, or any powerful oils that you work with. Your intentions need to be in alignment with the evoking of the masculine and feminine presence of God to come into you. Make this your sincere prayer as you speak aloud the aspects of God that you are invoking. Remember the power of ren. When you name something you give it form. From now on you will invoke these aspects of God every morning upon waking, every night upon falling asleep, and every time you make love. This has to be a given.

Anoint all seven chakras paying special attention to the awakening of the threefold flame gateways held within the third eye (wisdom), heart (love), and womb/hara (power). This is a beautiful ceremony to perform for one another. Play some music that reflects the holy moment, and drench the space in sacred candlelight.

Holy Matrimony

The Sacrament of Holy Matrimony is what you have been truly doing. It is the sacred act of hieros gamos, the reunion of fire and water, masculine and feminine, night and day, yin and yang, and every pair of opposites found within duality.

Communion

The Sacrament of Communion is one of the most holy ceremonies as well as the most important as it commemorates the Last Supper. Through this sacrament we are led step by step to the purpose of our earthly lives—union with the Divine. During communion the faithful are made one with God and each other by receiving the body and blood of Christ under the earthly forms of bread and wine. However, in the gnostic tradition it is not *only* the body and blood of Christ but rather the body of Sophia and the blood of the Logos. This reunion with the Divine can only come about through the reunion of the Sophia within us all and the Logos—the love and light of God.

Through your sacred union process practice the ritual of communion at the beginning of every ten-day cycle, which I will explain a little further on. Use the traditional symbols of bread and red wine, or water, for your ritual. Bread is a symbol for the body of the feminine, the Holy Sophia, the chalice, the Holy Grail, the vessel, and the alchemical container. Wine is a symbol for the blood of the masculine, the light/love of the Logos, and the focused blade of alchemical spiritual fire. Bring them together in your ceremonial cup. Soak the bread in the wine; see, smell, sense, feel, and taste the reunion. As you consume the sacrament, feel the energies submerge into your being and pierce your heart. Herein lies the true meaning of communion.

Confession

Originally the confession of error (sin) was done aloud as it still is in most Catholic churches. But even when whispered the power of confession is taken to a whole new level. The spoken whisper relates to the magical power of words and sound as embodied in the idea of the Hindu mantras and the Christian Logos, the word. Jesus Christ imparted the power of forgiving the sins to the apostles by blowing or whispering upon them as the Holy Spirit (described in John 20:21–23).

When entering conscious communication with your beloved be aware that whispered words spoken slowly and deliberately between you have the power to release you of error, especially if you are communicating from a place of wounding or agitation. It is important that you open a regular space for confession so that you can release any buildup of tension and emotional charge as well as any events that play out in the dream/sleep state. Just because we are asleep doesn't mean that these energies cannot interfere with the sacred union process, especially if they are of a sexual or darker nature. Our partners will absolutely sense the change in our energy and know on some level that something has happened. So the wise and true thing to do is to share immediately, just as you would if these events were happening in the awake state.

Ordination

Ordination is the rite of the Christian church for the commissioning of priests and priestesses. The ceremony consists of a laying on of hands on the top of the head of the priest or priestess. Symbolically the laying on of hands transmits a spark of the spirit into the initiate, just as a burning candle can impart its flame to an unlit candle. Through ordination then, an uninterrupted chain is established, which stretches all the way back to the origin of the sacred lineage.

For our purposes ordination is quite simply the sharing of this sacred work with other couples. Use all that you have learned and experienced along the way to help catalyze healing in others who may be experiencing sexual suppression, emotional wounding, and layers of builtup resentment and distrust.

The Anointing of the Sick

The anointing of the sick is a practice of most, if not all religions. It is an extremely ancient and universal ritual. The sacrament is often administered by a priest who uses oil to anoint the person's forehead or other parts of the body while reciting certain prayers. It is believed to bring comfort, peace, courage, and even the forgiveness of sins, if the person is unable to speak.

Through the sacrament a gift of the Holy Spirit is given that renews confidence and faith in God and strengthens us against temptations of discouragement, despair, and anguish at the thought of death and the struggle of death. The sacrament nourishes the person and keeps them from losing faith in God's love, truth, and presence.

In my deepest, innermost knowing I believe that those of us who move through the sacred union process will be able to harness and use the gifts of the Holy Spirit and be able to perform such ceremonies as these. My faith tells me that immense waves of love shall emanate from within the hearts of those who have reunified and that their presence alone shall have the power to heal all bitterness and hardness of heart. Even their glance will bring hope and faith in abundance to the souls of all humanity.

For our purposes please practice the anointing of the sick should one of you fall ill or if any life-form should cross your path that is in pain or in need. Remember the sacraments are invocations of grace.

They should not be seen as duties but rather delightful gifts to bestow upon the world.

The Sacred Vows

And finally here is the last piece of the puzzle: the soul-braiding process.

The merging of your ten light bodies happens by a process known as soul braiding. This happens as a result of weaving together the light bodies in meditation and by the spoken sacred vows of your soul. Before you begin the sacred union process drop in to the innermost core of your being as you feel into the marriage vows that you are choosing to commit to. Instead of the priest or registrar speaking out your marriage vows as in a traditional ceremony, you instead choose them and speak them to one another. When I took the time to do this I spent a beautiful leisurely few days truly feeling into the noble qualities of the presence and commitment that I was yearning to give to my beloved. I took this time to write from my queenly heart all the powerful oaths and vows that I was hungry to live by. Even the process of writing these vows filled me with an energy that expanded my consciousness and heart. When I spoke to my beloved about the process he said how much he loved the process of really feeling into his sovereign masculinity. Here is an example of some of the vows that I made.

> *I, Anaiya Sophia, vow to my beloved king and husband
> [add beloved's name here] for the rest of my life and
> existence:*
>
> *to stand beside you, planted firmly in the ground upon
> which we stand*
> *to love and honor you*
> *to love you as God loves us*
> *to hold your heart as our child*

> *to always love and welcome God as the third being*
> *to stand in the fire with you*
> *to hold our relationship within the sacred circle*
> *to love you through all that life presents to us*
> *to fill our lives with happiness, joy, and laughter.*

Because I consistently work with the sacred meaning of numbers, I chose thirty-three vows in total. For our purposes the ritual goes like this: Every morning and night as you come together in meditation you invoke one of your ten bodies. Starting with the physical body and following the same flow that I used in chapter 8, you will take it in turns to speak your vows *from and to* that particular body. When you receive the vows from your partner, you consciously listen *from within* the particular body you are working with as you take the sound current of your beloved's voice and guide its essence deep into the heart of that body. In summary one of you whispers their vows with full presence and nobility while the other receives the vows into his or her awareness by the art of listening and then by energetically guiding the vows into the relevant dimensional space. After you have completed all your vows the other person says his or hers.

Because we are working with a thirty-day period you would repeat this ten-day cycle three times. For the first round be aware that your vows are coated and wrapped in the energies of your sexuality. For the second round be aware that your vows are coated and wrapped in the energies of your heart. Finally, for the third round be aware that your vows are coated and wrapped in the energies of your soul.

My final gift to you as you enter the bridal chamber are these last words and the reminder to not even take this book into the sacred space, for your guide is now the mystery itself.

Behold the rites of love. Follow the path that has been laid out for you, and you will find what you seek. Once you have found it, you must share it with the world and fulfill the three sacred promises that you made.

* *The first promise is to God, your Mother and Father. It represents your most divine destiny and purpose, what you have come to accomplish in the image of your Creators. It is the reason for your incarnation, the purest intention of your soul. This promise is found within your wisdom flame and consciousness.*

* *The second promise is to your soul half and the soul family within which you were created and that you will belong to through eternity. It represents your relationship to each of the 144 souls in your family—how you have agreed to assist them in their mission and they in yours. This promise is found within your love flame and heart.*

* *The third promise is to yourself. It represents how you desire to learn and grow and love within the context of this incarnation. This promise is found within your flame of power and your sexuality.*

Our truth has been in darkness for too long.
Amor vincit omnia. *Love conquers all.*

ANAIYA SOPHIA

I move forward with trust and consciousness.

BIBLIOGRAPHY

Barks, Coleman, trans. *Rumi: The Book Of Love: Poems of Ecstasy and Longing.* New York: HarperCollins Publishing, 2003.

Deida, David. *The Way of the Superior Man: A Spiritual Guide to Mastering the Challenges of Women, Work, and Sexual Desire.* Boulder, Colo.: Sounds True, 1997.

DeRohan, Ceanne. *The Right Use of Will.* 8 vols. Santa Fe, N.Mex.: Four Winds Publication, 1986–1989.

Faulkner, Raymond, trans. *The Egyptian Book of the Dead: The Book of Going Forth by Day,* 2nd ed. San Francisco: Chronicle Books, 2000.

Gibran, Kahlil. *The Collected Works: Everyman's Library.* New York: Alfred A. Knopf, 2007.

Houston, Jean. *The Passion of Isis and Osiris: A Gateway to Transcendent Love.* New York: Wellspring/Ballantine, 1998.

Leloup, Jean-Yves, trans. *The Gospel of Mary Magdalene.* Rochester, Vt.: Inner Traditions, 2002.

———. *The Gospel of Philip.* Rochester, Vt.: Inner Traditions, 2004.

———. *The Gospel of Thomas.* Rochester, Vt.: Inner Traditions, 2005.

Ludwig, Emil. *Of Life and Love.* New York: The Philosophical Library, 1945.

McGowan, Kathleen. *The Book of Love.* New York: Touchstone, Simon & Schuster, 2009.

Miller, Rosamonde Ikshvàku. "Ritual of the Bridal Chamber: The Gnostic Mystery of the Eucharist." Church of Gnosis http://gnosticsanctuary.org/eucharist.html.

Miller, Rosamonde Ikshvàku, trans. and ed. "An Excerpt from *The Testament of Miriam of Magdala.*" 2005, www.marymagdaleneshrine.org/egyptian.swf.

Mueller, Joan, trans. *Clare of Assisi: The Letters to Agnes.* Collegeville, Minn.: Liturgical Press, 2003.

Prakasha, Anaiya Aon (Anaiya Sophia). *Pilgrimage of Love: A Tale of Romance, Heartbreak and Meeting "The One."* Self-published using Lulu.com, 2011.

Prakasha, Padma Aon. *The Nine Eyes of Light: Ascension Keys from Egypt.* Berkeley, Calif.: North Atlantic Books, 2010.

Prakasha, Padma Aon, and Anaiya Aon Prakasha (Anaiya Sophia). *Womb Wisdom: Awakening the Creative and Forgotten Powers of the Feminine.* Rochester, Vt: Destiny Books, 2011.

Robinson, James M., ed. *The Nag Hammadi Library: The Definitive Translation of the Gnostic Scriptures Complete in One Volume.* New York: Harper San Francisco, 1990.

St. Cloud, Terri. *Her White Tree.* Accokeek, Md.: Bone Sigh Arts, 2011.

Stockham, Alice Bunker. *Karezza, Ethics of Marriage.* Chicago: Stockham Publishing, 1903.

Williamson, Marianne. "The Romantic Mysteries." January 9, 2012, http://blog.marianne.com/journal/index.php.

Weor, Samael Aun, trans. *The Gnostic Bible: The Pistis Sophia Unveiled.* New York: Glorian Publishing, 2011.

CDS

All CD's have been mixed and produced by Elwyn Lear. For more information contact elwynlear@googlemail.com.

Sophia, Anaiya. *Bridal Chamber.* 2013 by Anaiya Sophia.

———. *Womb.* 2012 by Anaiya Sophia.

———. *Wounds of Love.* 2012 by Anaiya Sophia.

Sophia, Anaiya and Luc Tibor Erdos, *Sacred Union.* 2013 by Anaiya Sophia.

INDEX

Page numbers in *italics* refer to illustrations.